Advances in
Breast Cancer Management

Cancer Treatment and Research

Steven T. Rosen, M.D., *Series Editor*

Goldstein, L.J., Ozols, R. F. (eds.): Anticancer Drug Resistance. Advances in Molecular and Clinical Research. 1994. ISBN 0-7923-2836-1.

Hong, W.K., Weber, R.S. (eds.): Head and Neck Cancer. Basic and Clinical Aspects. 1994. ISBN 0-7923-3015-3.

Thall, P.F. (ed): Recent Advances in Clinical Trial Design and Analysis. 1995. ISBN 0-7923-3235-0.

Buckner, C. D. (ed): Technical and Biological Components of Marrow Transplantation. 1995. ISBN 0-7923-3394-2.

Winter, J.N. (ed.): Blood Stem Cell Transplantation. 1997. ISBN 0-7923-4260-7.

Muggia, F.M. (ed): Concepts, Mechanisms, and New Targets for Chemotherapy. 1995. ISBN 0-7923-3525-2.

Klastersky, J. (ed): Infectious Complications of Cancer. 1995. ISBN 0-7923-3598-8.

Kurzrock, R., Talpaz, M. (eds): Cytokines: Interleukins and Their Receptors. 1995. ISBN 0-7923-3636-4.

Sugarbaker, P. (ed): Peritoneal Carcinomatosis: Drugs and Diseases. 1995. ISBN 0-7923-3726-3.

Sugarbaker, P. (ed): Peritoneal Carcinomatosis: Principles of Management. 1995. ISBN 0-7923-3727-1.

Dickson, R.B., Lippman, M.E. (eds.): Mammary Tumor Cell Cycle, Differentiation and Metastasis. 1995. ISBN 0-7923-3905-3.

Freireich, E.J, Kantarjian, H. (eds.): Molecular Genetics and Therapy of Leukemia. 1995. ISBN 0-7923-3912-6.

Cabanillas, F., Rodriguez, M.A. (eds.): Advances in Lymphoma Research. 1996. ISBN 0-7923-3929-0.

Miller, A.B. (ed.): Advances in Cancer Screening. 1996. ISBN 0-7923-4019-1.

Hait , W.N. (ed.): Drug Resistance. 1996. ISBN 0-7923-4022-1.

Pienta, K.J. (ed.): Diagnosis and Treatment of Genitourinary Malignancies. 1996. ISBN 0-7923-4164-3.

Arnold, A.J. (ed.): Endocrine Neoplasms. 1997. ISBN 0-7923-4354-9.

Pollock, R.E. (ed.): Surgical Oncology. 1997. ISBN 0-7923-9900-5.

Verweij, J., Pinedo, H.M., Suit, H.D. (eds.): Soft Tissue Sarcomas: Present Achievements and Future Prospects. 1997. ISBN 0-7923-9913-7.

Walterhouse, D.O., Cohn, S. L. (eds.): Diagnostic and Therapeutic Advances in Pediatric Oncology. 1997. ISBN 0-7923-9978-1.

Mittal, B.B., Purdy, J.A., Ang, K.K. (eds.): Radiation Therapy. 1998. ISBN 0-7923-9981-1.

Foon, K.A., Muss, H.B. (eds.): Biological and Hormonal Therapies of Cancer. 1998. ISBN 0-7923-9997-8.

Ozols, R.F. (ed.): Gynecologic Oncology. 1998. ISBN 0-7923-8070-3.

Noskin, G. A. (ed.): Management of Infectious Complications in Cancer Patients. 1998. ISBN 0-7923-8150-5

Bennett, C. L. (ed.): Cancer Policy. 1998. ISBN 0-7923-8203-X

Benson, A. B. (ed.): Gastrointestinal Oncology. 1998. ISBN 0-7923-8205-6

Tallman, M.S. , Gordon, L.I. (eds.): Diagnostic and Therapeutic Advances in Hematologic Malignancies. 1998. ISBN 0-7923-8206-4

von Gunten, C.F. (ed.): Palliative Care and Rehabilitation of Cancer Patients. 1999. ISBN 0-7923-8525-X

Burt, R.K., Brush, M.M. (eds): Advances in Allogeneic Hematopoietic Stem Cell Transplantation. 1999. ISBN 0-7923-7714-1

Angelos, P. (ed): Ethical Issues in Cancer Patient Care 2000. ISBN 0-7923-7726-5

Gradishar, W.J., Wood, W.C. (eds): Advances in Breast Cancer Management. 2000. ISBN 0-7923-7890-3

ADVANCES IN BREAST CANCER MANAGEMENT

edited by

William J. Gradishar, M.D.

Associate Professor of Medicine
Director, Breast Medical Oncology
Division of Hematology/Oncology
Robert H. Lurie Comprehensive Cancer Center
Northwestern University Medical School, USA

and

William C. Wood, M.D.

Joseph Brown Whitehead Professor and Chairman
Department of Surgery
Emory University School of Medicine, USA

KLUWER ACADEMIC PUBLISHERS
Boston / Dordrecht / London

Distributors for North, Central and South America:
Kluwer Academic Publishers
101 Philip Drive
Assinippi Park
Norwell, Massachusetts 02061 USA

Distributors for all other countries:
Kluwer Academic Publishers Group
Distribution Centre
Post Office Box 322
3300 AH Dordrecht, THE NETHERLANDS

Library of Congress Cataloging-in-Publication Data

Table of Contents

List of Author's Titles/Addresses

Melody A. Cobleigh, M.D.
Professor of Medicine
Director, Comprehensive Breast Center
Rush-Presbyterian-St. Luke's Medical Center
1725 West Harrison Street
Suite 821
Chicago, IL 60612

Michael Crump, M.D.
Associate Professor of Medicine
Toronto-Sunnybrook Regional Cancer Center
2075 Bayview Avenue
Toronto, Ontario M4N 3M5
Canada

Bernard Fisher, M.D.
Distinguish Service Professor
University of Pittsburgh
Allegheny University of the Health Sciences
Four Allegheny Center
Suite 602
Pittsburgh, PA 15212-5234

William J. Gradishar, M.D.
Associate Professor of Medicine
Director, Breast Medical Oncology
Northwestern University Medical School
Division of Hematology/Oncology
Robert H. Lurie Comprehensive Cancer Center
676 North St. Clair Street
Suite 850
Chicago, IL 60611-2927

Armando E. Giuliano, M.D.
Chief of Surgical Oncology
John Wayne Cancer Institute at St. John's Health Center
Clinical Professor of Surgery
UCLA School of Medicine
John Wayne Cancer Institute
2200 Santa Monica Boulevard
Santa Monica, CA 90404

Philip J. Haigh, M.D., F.R.C.S.(C.)
Clinical Fellow
John Wayne Cancer Institute
Surgical Oncology
2200 Santa Monica Boulevard
Santa Monica, CA 90404

Gottfried Konecny, M.D.
Post-Graduate Research Fellow
Division of Hematology/Oncology
Department of Medicine
University of California, Los Angeles
11-934 Factor Building
10833 LeConte Avenue
Los Angeles, CA 90095-1678

Eleftherios P. Mamounas, M.D.
Clinical Assistant Professor in Surgery
Case Western Reserve University
Mt. Sinai Center for Breast Health
26900 Cedar Road
Suite 310
Beachwood, OH 44122

Yago Nieto, M.D.
Instructor
University of Colorado Health Sciences Center
Bone Marrow Transplant Program
4200 East 9th Avenue
Denver, CO 80262

Ruth M. O'Regan, M.D.
Instructor
Northwestern University Medical School
Division of Hematology/Oncology
Robert H. Lurie Comprehensive Cancer Center
676 North St. Clair Street
Suite 850
Chicago, IL 60611-2927

Mark D. Pegram, M.D.
Adjunct Assistant Professor
Division of Hematology/Oncology
Department of Medicine
University of California, Los Angeles
11-934 Factor Building
10833 LeConte Avenue
Los Angeles, CA 90095-1678

Kathleen Pritchard, M.D.
Professor of Medicine
Toronto-Sunnybrook Regional Cancer Center
2075 Bayview Avenue
Toronto, Ontario M4N 3M5
Canada

Peter M. Ravdin, M.D.
Associate Professor of Medicine
University of Texas Health Science Center at San Antonio
7703 Floyd Curl Drive, Room 5
San Antonio, TX 78284-6200

Abram Recht, M.D.
Associate Professor of Medicine
Harvard Medical School and
Beth Israel Deaconess Medical Center
Department of Radiation Oncology
330 Brookline Avenue
Boston, MA 02215-5491

Elizabeth J. Shpall, M.D.
Professor of Medicine
University of Colorado Health Sciences Center
Bone Marrow Transplant Program
4200 East 9th Avenue
Denver, CO 80262

Dennis J. Slamon, M.D., Ph.D.
Professor and Chief
Division of Hematology/Oncology
Department of Medicine
University of California, Los Angeles
11-934 Factor Building
10833 LeConte Avenue
Los Angeles, CA 90095-1678

William C. Wood, M.D.
Joseph Brown Whitehead Professor and Chairman
Clinical Director, Cancer Center
Emory University School of Medicine
Department of Surgery
1364 Clifton Road, N.E.
Suite B206
Atlanta, GA 30322-1104

Preface

The optimal management of breast cancer patients relies on the expertise of a team of medical specialists including radiologists, surgeons, radiation therapists and medical oncologists. Much of the progress in breast cancer management made over the last several years reflects the translation of observations made in the laboratory to the clinic. Critically evaluating the impact of new treatment approaches relies on a commitment to well-designed clinical trials.

In this volume, *Advances in Breast Cancer Management*, a renowned group of breast cancer experts have been asked to provide their perspective on management issues that directly effect patients on a day-to-day basis. Dr. Melody Cobleigh discusses the consequences of estrogen deprivation and the ways of ameliorating secondary symptoms and the potential long-term morbidity. Drs. Haigh and Guiliano review the sentinel lymph node biopsy technique including results from their extensive experience. Dr. Abram Recht places into perspective the potential benefit of post-mastectomy radiotherapy and reviews recent trials that address this issue. Dr. Dennis Slamon takes from us from the laboratory to the clinic in explaining the development of Herceptin as a paradigm for therapy targeted to specific molecular characteristics of breast cancer tumor cells. Drs. Nieto, Shpall, Crump and Pritchard offer different perspectives on the future of high-dose chemotherapy with stem cell transplantation as a treatment for breast cancer patients. Drs. Mamounas and Fisher discuss the rationale for considering preoperative chemotherapy in patients with operable breast cancer and review the results from National Surgical Adjuvant Breast and Bowel Project randomized clinical trials that address the relative efficacy of this approach compared to standard, post-operative adjuvant chemotherapy. Dr. Peter Ravdin explains the power of meta-analysis techniques to evaluate the efficacy of adjuvant chemotherapy and endocrine treatment. He reviews the important findings from the most recent Oxford Overview analysis of randomized adjuvant therapy trials in early stage breast cancer. Finally, Dr. Ruth O'Regan provides an overview of the results from the recently completed tamoxifen prevention trials in women at increased risk of developing breast cancer.

We believe that the contributors to this volume have succeeded in providing the most recent data available on their respective topics. Furthermore they have offered us insight into where challenges remain in optimizing the care of breast cancer patients.

William J. Gradishar, MD
William C. Wood, MD

1

Managing Menopausal Problems

Melody A. Cobleigh, M.D.
Professor of Medicine
Rush-Presbyterian-St. Luke's Medical Center

INTRODUCTION

Breast cancer survivors often seek advice about menopausal problems from their oncologists. In addition, oncologists interact with colleagues about their patients' menopausal issues. For these reasons, it is important that oncologists be knowledgeable about the effects of hormone replacement therapy (HRT) on overall health. And the need for up-to-the-minute information is intensified by the plethora of new drugs, the greater frequency with which pharmaceutical companies market directly to the public, and the increasing interest of patients in alternative therapies.

W.J. Gradishar and W.C. Wood (eds.), ADVANCES IN BREAST CANCER MANAGEMENT, Copyright © 2000. Kluwer Academic Publishers, Boston. All rights reserved.

GENERAL CONSIDERATIONS

Changes in Metabolism

One of the most important lessons we can teach our menopausal patients (whether menopause is naturally or chemotherapeutically induced) is that unless they eat less or exercise more they will gain weight. Women lose fat-free mass after menopause. They also tend to exercise less during leisure time and to experience greater increases in fat mass, fasting insulin levels, and waist-to-hip ratio. Breast cancer survivors often blame the changing shapes of their bodies on tamoxifen although double blind, randomized trials show no difference in weight for placebo-vs-tamoxifen-treated patients.[1]

Simply put, postmenopausal women burn fewer calories at rest than do premenopausal women, suggesting that estrogen helps control weight.[2] The suggestion is supported by the postmenopausal estrogen-progesterone prevention (PEPI) trial. In this double blind, randomized study, women who received a placebo gained significantly more weight than those treated with estrogen.[3] Evidence that weight gain is a significant health concern for breast cancer survivors comes from the Nurses' Health Study, which found that weight gain after menopause increases breast cancer incidence and mortality among women who do not take HRT.[4]

Vasomotor Instability

The most common reason Western women seek hormonal intervention at menopause is vasomotor symptoms. As many as 85% experience perimenopausal hot flashes and night sweats, and HRT reduces the number of hot flashes by 80% after one month of treatment.[5] Women who undergo premature menopause as a consequence of chemotherapy are more symptomatic from vasomotor instability than their naturally menopausal counterparts, and they are likely to seek medical intervention to alleviate their discomfort. Among breast cancer survivors who had heard or read about HRT, 51% had talked to their doctor about it after their diagnosis,[6] and 31% were willing to take HRT under medical supervision.

In Southeast Asia, vasomotor symptoms are less frequent (20-40%).[7] One reason for the difference may be the difficulty of recognizing symptoms of thermoregulatory imbalance in a warm climate; however, another important explanation may be that Asian diets, which are often rich in phytoestrogens, ameliorate hot flashes.

Nonhormonal remedies for hot flashes include clonidine, which decreases the frequency and severity of hot flashes (Table 1). Although statistically significant, the clinical benefit is modest and may be achieved at the expense of constipation, dry mouth, and drowsiness. Another alpha$_2$-adrenoceptor agonist, methyldopa, reduces the frequency of hot flashes significantly, but can also be associated with unpleasant side effects (tiredness and dry mouth). Bellergal S is effective. Bellergal works in the short run, but is ineffective after eight weeks. Vitamin E and dong quai (*Angelica polymorpha* a plant of the carrot family) are ineffective. In an open label study, venlafaxine reduced symptoms in 58% of women.[8] A double blind, placebo controlled, randomized trial is under way.

Progestational agents for the relief of hot flashes: Progestational agents are more effective than placebo in relieving hot flashes (Table 2). Physicians seem more comfortable prescribing progestogens than estrogens to relieve vasomotor symptoms in breast cancer survivors. However, the effect of progesterone on normal and malignant breast cells is unknown. In striking contrast to the endometrium, where progesterone is associated with reduced proliferation, mitotic activity in breast epithelium peaks during days 23-25 of the menstrual cycle. This is shortly after the progesterone peak and the second estradiol peak, suggesting that progesterone, or possibly the combination of estrogen and progesterone, is responsible.[9, 10, 11] Progestins have been implicated in the development of breast cancer in humans[12] as well as in experimental animals[13, 14, 15] and laboratory cell cultures.[16, 17, 18]

Table 1. Nonhormonal Alternatives to HRT For Relief of Hot Flashes

| | | | % Reduction in Hot Flashes | |
Author	No. of Patients	Medication	Treatment	Placebo
Nesheim[19]	40	Methyldopa 250 mg 1 bid; ↑ to 2 bid if no success	65* (45-75)	38 (0-59)
Bergmans[20]	66	Bellergal Retard 1 bid	75	68
Lebherz[21]	72	Bellergal S 1 bid	60	22
Goldberg[22]	110	Clonidine patch (0.1 mg/day)	44	27
Barton[23]	125	Vitamin E 400 IU bid	25	22
Hirata[24]	71	dong quai 4.5 g daily	33	29

* Significantly better than placebo.

Table 2. Placebo-Controlled Randomized Trials of Progestational Agents For Relief of Vasomotor Symptoms

Author	No. of Patients	Medication	% Reduction in Hot Flashes	
			Treatment	Placebo
Loprinzi[19]	80	MA	73	26
Morrison[26]	34	MPA	68	20
Albrecht[27]	6	MPA	87	25
Schiff[28]	32	MPA	74	26
Bullock[29]	57 MPA 12 Placebo	MPA	90	25

Interactions between progestational agents and tamoxifen have not been studied in breast cancer survivors. Clinically, the combination of progestins and tamoxifen is less effective than tamoxifen alone in metastatic breast cancer.[30] Further concerns are raised by the finding that progesterone, given for only one week per month, reverses the protective effect of tamoxifen in a rat mammary carcinoma model.[31]

Selective estrogen receptor modulators (SERMs): Raloxifene does not alleviate and may exacerbate hot flashes. In a randomized, controlled trial the incidence of hot flashes was 23% in the placebo group and 26% in the group receiving 60 mg of raloxifene.[32] Women with "serious postmenopausal symptoms were excluded from the trial. Leg cramps were more common among women treated with raloxifene (2.6%) than among those receiving placebo (0.7%). Tamoxifen significantly increases the incidence of hot flashes.[33]

HRT and tamoxifen: Breast cancer survivors who suffer severe menopausal symptoms are offered HRT and tamoxifen at the Royal Marsden Hospital.[34] Tamoxifen and HRT appeared to interact favorably in a small subset of participants in the British breast cancer prevention trial.[35] The combination caused a reduction in serum cholesterol, an increase in bone mineral density, and no adverse change in coagulation factors. Participants in the Italian breast cancer prevention trial were allowed to continue HRT along with placebo or tamoxifen. Italian researchers found a statistically significant reduction in breast cancer among those who received HRT plus tamoxifen compared with those who received HRT plus placebo.[36] Neither the British nor the Italian group has studied whether HRT relieves hot flashes in women taking tamoxifen. This is the primary objective of the Eastern Cooperative Oncology Group HRT/tamoxifen trial.

Maintaining Bone Health

Bone mineral density decreases rapidly during the first five years after natural menopause. Osteoporotic fractures are an important cause of morbidity in old age and affect 50% of women over age 50.[37] Breast cancer survivors are at particular risk because of chemotherapy-induced premature menopause. A prospective study of women who suffered chemical castration from adjuvant chemotherapy showed that bone loss was 9.5% at the lumbar spine and 4.6% at the femoral neck after just two years.[38] Thus, it is important to maintain the bone health of postmenopausal women, and several strategies are needed.

Diet: Postmenopausal women need 1500 mg of calcium daily. A serving of dairy products such as a glass of milk or a portion of yogurt contains 200 mg of calcium, so supplements are often necessary. Calcium citrate is better absorbed than calcium carbonate. Vitamin D (700 units per day) is also important, particularly for individuals who are deprived of sunlight. This simple dietary intervention has resulted in reductions of 30%-70% in fracture rates over two to four years.[39]

Exercise: Weight-bearing exercise such as walking, jogging, or aerobics should be performed for at least 30 minutes three times per week.

Assessment: A woman's height should be measured not only to enable the physician to accurately calculate body surface area for treatment purposes but as a baseline for yearly follow-up of skeletal health. It is not sufficient to ask the patient how tall she is because she may be unaware that she has already lost height from osteoporosis. A baseline bone mineral density, repeated every two years, will show osteopenia before irreparable damage has occurred.

Medication for prevention of osteoporosis: HRT has been shown to prevent osteoporosis in a randomized, placebo-controlled trial.[40] Participants assigned to placebo lost an average of 1.8% and 1.7%, respectively, of spine and hip bone mineral density after three years. Those assigned to active treatment gained bone mineral density, ranging from 3.5% to 5% at the spine and averaging 1.7% at the hip.

Tamoxifen significantly reduces bone loss in postmenopausal breast cancer survivors.[41] A randomized, controlled trial showed that raloxifene protected bone density significantly more than placebo over a two-year period.[42]

(Information on fracture prevention is not yet available.) Participants were postmenopausal and did not have osteoporosis. Breast cancer survivors were excluded, as were women with "serious" postmenopausal symptoms or abnormal uterine bleeding. Although the FDA has approved raloxifene (60 mg per day) for prevention of osteoporosis, the drug has not been adequately studied in women with a history of breast cancer.

A randomized, placebo-controlled trial showed that alendronate protected bone significantly more than placebo over a three-year period.[43] Participants were postmenopausal and did not have osteoporosis, and women with major upper gastrointestinal diseases were excluded. Another randomized trial showed that alendronate with HRT was more effective than alendronate alone.[44] The FDA has approved alendronate (5 mg per day) for prevention of osteoporosis.

Medication for treating osteoporosis: The reduction in the rate of osteoporotic fracture in HRT users ranges between 30% and 60%.[45,46] A randomized, placebo-controlled trial showed that alendronate progressively increased bone mass in the spine, hip, and total body while reducing the incidence of vertebral fractures and height loss in postmenopausal women with osteoporosis.[47] The FDA has approved alendronate (10 mg per day) for treatment of osteoporosis. A 19% reduction in fractures at the hip site, and lower radius almost reached statistical significance at a mean of four years of treatment in a tamoxifen breast cancer prevention trial.[33]

Cardiovascular Health

Unless women understand that they are vulnerable to coronary artery disease (CAD), they will be unwilling to make the personal changes necessary to prevent cardiovascular illness. The most important health-related behaviors are to avoid smoking, eat a healthy diet, and exercise moderately to help control weight.

Diet and dietary supplements: A balanced diet that is low in saturated fat helps control blood lipid levels. Observational studies suggest that consumption of 400-800 units of vitamin E daily exerts a protective effect against CAD.[48]

Decades ago, the relationship between homocysteinuria and premature vascular occlusive disease was discovered in patients with a rare inborn error of metabolism. The discovery led to the hypothesis that elevated blood homocysteine levels may be a risk factor for CAD. Dietary supplementation with folate alone or folate plus vitamin B6 and vitamin B12 reduces homocysteine levels. Epidemiologic information suggests that supplemental intake of folate and vitamin B6 above the current recommended dietary allowance is important for primary prevention of CAD among women. The adjusted odds ratio for CAD among women who consume a daily multiple vitamin is .76.[49] Supplementation is especially important among women who regularly consume alcoholic beverages. In this group the adjusted odds ratio for CAD among those who take a multiple vitamin supplement daily is .22.

Premature menopause: CAD is an insidious but potentially fatal consequence of menopausal estrogen decline. Because the treatment of breast cancer in young women can precipitate premature menopause, its ovarian toxicity is a matter of serious concern. Even though adjuvant chemotherapy causes premature ovarian failure,[50] it is prescribed more often now, based on favorable outcomes for women with small invasive but node-negative disease.[51,52,53] However, review of the role of premature menopause in CAD found an increased risk in women with early menopause.[54] Evidence that HRT can reduce this effect of early menopause comes from the Nurses' Health Study, in which women who underwent surgical menopause and received HRT had a significantly lower risk of cardiovascular disease than those with surgical menopause who did not receive HRT.[55]

Most node-negative women are cured of breast cancer, and death from non-neoplastic conditions is common. Moreover, cardiovascular disease is the most common cause of noncancer deaths even in patients who did not receive chemotherapy and thus did not undergo premature menopause.[56] As more node-negative women receive adjuvant chemotherapy, we must acknowledge the possibility that early chemotherapy-mediated gains in survival from breast cancer may be overshadowed by later increases in mortality from cardiovascular and osteoporotic events. That is, women may survive their breast cancers, only to succumb to more common but delayable afflictions. The latest meta-analysis does not yet suggest, with 15 years of follow-up, that there is an increase in non-breast cancer mortality in women who have received chemotherapy.[57] However, node-negative women represent the overwhelming majority in the analysis, and therefore breast cancer mortality may obscure such an effect.

The National Surgical Adjuvant Breast Project B-20 trial showed that chemotherapy regimens that do not cause ovarian failure are useful as adjuvant therapy.[58] Premenopausal, node-negative, estrogen receptor-positive patients benefited significantly from tamoxifen plus methotrexate, 5-fluorouracil, and leucovorin, a regimen that does not cause premature ovarian failure. This regimen compared favorably with tamoxifen plus cyclophosphamide, methotrexate, and 5-fluorouracil, a chemotherapy regimen known for significant ovarian toxicity.

Aspirin: Aspirin is an option for prevention in postmenopausal women at high risk for cardiovascular disease. High-risk subjects include those with acute or prior myocardial infarction, a history of stroke or transient ischemic attack, unstable or stable angina, vascular surgery, angioplasty, atrial fibrillation, valvular heart disease, or peripheral vascular disease. Treatment with 75-325 mg per day offered significant protection against myocardial infarction, stroke, and death in a meta-analysis of randomized trials.[59]

The statins: Drug therapy for hypercholesterolemia, particularly for women, has remained controversial because of insufficient clinical evidence that treatment enhances survival; however, some reports showed important benefits. In the Scandinavian Simvastatin study, women randomly assigned to Simvastatin had an absolute 35% reduction in major coronary events compared with placebo-treated women.[60] Another placebo-controlled trial in healthy middle-aged women with average cholesterol and low-density lipoprotein-C and with below-average high-density lipoprotein-C levels showed that Lovastatin offered significant benefit in primary prevention of acute coronary events.[61]

Estrogen and SERMs: HRT reduces CAD significantly. Women who undergo natural menopause and take HRT experience a 30%-70% reduction in heart attack.[45,62,63] A randomized trial showed that 60 mg of raloxifene favorably altered biochemical markers of cardiovascular risk. It reduced low-density lipoprotein, fibrinogen, and lipoprotein(a) significantly more than placebo over a six-month period in healthy postmenopausal women.[64] Information on prevention of myocardial infarction is not yet available. Breast cancer survivors were excluded from the trial, as were women with "serious" postmenopausal symptoms or abnormal uterine bleeding. Although HRT had no effect on fibrinogen and raised triglycerides significantly, it proved superior to raloxifene in raising high-density lipoprotein and in lowering lipoprotein(a) and PAI-1.

The effects of SERMs on lipid profiles are remarkably similar (Table 3). It is therefore notable that no decrease in cardiovascular events has been observed in the Oxford overview analysis of adjuvant tamoxifen trials.[65] This is not surprising, since the beneficial effect on atherogenesis attributable to alteration of lipoproteins in primates accounts for only about one-third of the overall benefit seen with HRT.[66]

Table 3. Effects of SERMs on Blood Lipids

Lipid	Good Change	HRT[63]	Tamoxifen[67]	Raloxifene[64]	Toremifene[65]	Soy phytoestrogens[48]
LDL-C	↓	↓	↓	↓	↓	↓
HDL-C	↑	↑	↔	↔	↑	↑
Triglycerides	↓	↑	↑	↔	↔	↓
Lp(a)	↓	↓	↓	↓	↓	
Apo A-I	↑	↑	↔	↔	↑	↑
Apo B			↓	↓	↓	
PAI-1		↓		↔		
Fibrinogen	↓	↔	↔[69]	↓		

Soybean phytoestrogens: Soybean phytoestrogens have the same beneficial effects as conjugated equine estrogen (CEE) on plasma lipid and lipoprotein concentrations in postmenopausal primates, except for their effect on triglycerides and apo A-1, which is more favorable.[70] In addition to their lipid-altering effects, soy phytoestrogens, like estrogen, mediate favorable effects on coronary arteries directly. They cause vasodilatation and reduce uptake of lipid in the intima of the coronary artery.[70]

Alzheimer's Disease

The most recent meta-analysis of case-controlled and cohort studies found a 29% reduction in risk of dementia among estrogen users.[71] However, the findings of the studies were heterogeneous, and the authors advised awaiting results of the Women's Health Initiative before prescribing HRT for this indication.

Conspicuously missing in discussions about SERMs is whether they are agonists or antagonists for the brain. Long-term studies of cognitive function in women who are treated chronically with these agents will be important to understand this important interaction. Meanwhile, the increase in hot flashes, a centrally mediated effect that is associated with some SERMs, is cause for concern.

Endometrium and Vagina

Soybean phytoestrogens are not uterotrophic,[70] nor is raloxifene.[32] Tamoxifen stimulates the endometrium, and women who take it for five years have a 1% incidence of endometrial carcinoma. These cancers are stage I and curable by hysterectomy when women are carefully followed by their gynecologists.[33]

Vaginal symptoms are common among breast cancer survivors.[6] Estrogen relieves these symptoms and has been approved by the FDA for treatment of atrophic vaginitis, but not for women with a history of breast cancer. Some physicians are more willing to prescribe vaginal estrogen-containing creams than oral estrogens, not realizing that vaginal administration according to the dose recommendation of the package insert raises serum estrogen levels 16- to 20-fold higher than oral administration of the same dose.[72,73,74]

A 1994 study evaluated low-dose conjugated estrogens (0.3 mg three times per week for six months). It revealed satisfactory relief of symptoms in 95% of cases. Vaginal maturation index improved significantly, and serum estrogen levels were unchanged. Endometrial biopsies revealed proliferation in only one case.[75]

An estradiol-releasing vaginal ring produced impressive relief of urogenital atrophy in 222 women.[76] The total dose os estradiol during a 12-week period was 0.8 mg. There was no significant change in plasma levels of sex hormone-binding globulin or estradiol. Estrone levels increased by about 300 pmol/L to about 900 pmol/L, but remained below the postmenopausal range (<1400 pmol/L). Endometrial thickness was not increased after six months of treatment in a subset of 30 women who were studied.

A prospective, randomized, open label trial compared a nonhormonal local bioadhesive vaginal moisturizer (Replens®) with vaginal estrogen cream (Premarin®).[77] Replens improved vaginal health, though to a lesser extent than did Premarin cream. Replens improved vaginal moisture, fluid volume, elasticity and pH despite a lack of cornification. Because the study did not include quality-of-life measures, it provides no evidence of how changes in the vagina correlated with symptom relief. If Replens is prescribed, it should be used three times per week for at least a month.

Coagulation

Raloxifene, according to the package insert, is contraindicated in women with active venous thromboembolic events or a history of such events, including deep vein thrombosis, pulmonary embolism, or retinal vein thrombosis. Tamoxifen also causes thrombophlebitis in about 1% of women who take it for five years. This complication is largely limited to postmenopausal women.[33]

Colon Cancer

Two prospective cohort studies showed that HRT reduced the incidence of colon cancer.[79,80] A third prospective study proved that fewer colon adenomas occurred in HRT users.[81] Of note is that colon cancer is a common second primary malignancy among node-negative breast cancer survivors.[56] Long-term follow-up of adjuvant tamoxifen studies shows no increase in colon cancer.

Breast Tissue

The best information about the effect of HRT on normal breast tissue comes from a longitudinal evaluation of surgically postmenopausal cynomolgus macaques.[82] These animals share 98% of their DNA with homo sapiens, and females are similar to women in their reproductive physiologic and anatomic features.

CEE has a mammotrophic effect on the mammary glands of macaques, resulting in greater thickness and epithelial hyperplasia. Combined continuous HRT has a greater effect than CEE alone. Combined HRT also causes down-regulation of both estrogen and progesterone receptors. Both CEE and combined continuous HRT cause increased proliferative activity as measured by Ki-67 staining.

Interpretation of mammograms: Concern has been raised about whether HRT may increase breast density thereby delaying the diagnosis of breast cancer. A prospective, blinded trial showed an upward shift in mammographic density for 24%, a downward shift in 12%, and no change in 63%. Baseline density was significantly correlated with risk of mammographic degradation. That is, women who had the least dense breast tissue on mammograms were most likely to experience a change that made their mammograms more difficult to interpret.[83] Women who experienced an upward shift in mammographic density on HRT were also likely to have breast pain.[84]

A nested case-control study of mammograms performed on 1,104 women, with radiologists blinded to the treatment regimen, showed that change was related to type of HRT. Women consuming no HRT, estrogen alone, cyclic estrogen plus progesterone, and continuous combined estrogen plus progesterone showed a 3.1, 4.7, 9.6, and 27.5% incidence of mammographic degradation, respectively.[85] The majority of these changes were considered "slight." Corresponding mammographic improvements occurred in 9.6, 12.5, 12.6, and 3.9%, respectively.

HRT and second breast cancers: Concern over HRT-induced new breast cancers must be addressed in any trial of replacement therapy for breast cancer survivors, especially because a personal history of breast cancer is a strong risk factor for subsequent development of primary breast cancer.[86] The annual incidence of new primary breast cancers among breast cancer survivors is 14 per 1000, compared with 2 per 1000 in the general population.[87] The association between HRT and risk of breast cancer remains controversial, although more than 50 studies and six meta-analyses have been published since 1980 (Table 4).

Collectively, the studies do not show a consistently increased risk of breast cancer among women who have ever used HRT. Studies that controlled for screening showed no difference in relative risk between cases and controls.[88] This suggests that a detection bias may be operating in some studies reporting an increased risk of breast cancer among HRT users. Importantly, low-dose CEE (0.625 mg daily) for several years did not appreciably increase the risk of breast cancer.

Table 4. Meta-Analyses of Breast Cancer Incidence Among HRT Users vs Non-Users

Author	Relative risk, Any use	95% Confidence interval, any use	Relative risk, Longer vs shorter
DuPont[89]	1.07	1.0 – 1.15	Results inconclusive
Steinberg[90]	1.0	Not stated	1.3 after 15 yrs*
Armstrong[91]	1.01	.95 – 1.08	No effect
Grady & Ernster[92]	No increase	Not stated	1.25
Sillero-Arenas[93]	1.06	1.0 – 1.12	Not stated
Colditz[94]	1.02	.93 – 1.12	Not stated

* 95% confidence interval 1.2-1.6.

Although having ever used HRT does not appear to substantially increase the risk of breast cancer, there remains a concern that selected subgroups will be adversely affected. For example, some studies have suggested that long-term use (10-15 years or more) increases the risk of breast cancer. Although the results are based on small numbers of cases (because relatively few women have used HRT for 15 or more years), the findings are of concern.

A possible confounding factor in these studies is the finding that consumption of alcohol while using HRT increases absorption of estrogen significantly (threefold).[95] Thus, it will be important to control for alcohol consumption in future analyses.

Although the preponderance of evidence shows that short-term use (<10 years) of HRT does not appear to cause breast cancer in healthy women, it is possible that women with a personal history of breast cancer may be more susceptible to tumor-promoting effects of estrogen. Tamoxifen reduces the risk of contralateral breast cancers in women with a history of breast cancer,[96] and it reduces the incidence of invasive breast cancer during short-term follow-up of high-risk women.[33] Thus, it is possible that tamoxifen administered with HRT may attenuate any potential cancer-promoting effect of estrogen on breast cells. Interestingly, the prognosis of breast cancer patients who received HRT before diagnosis is better than that of patients with no recorded exposure (Table 5).

Table 5. Relative Risk of Mortality from Breast Cancer Among HRT Users Compared With Never Users in Cohort Studies

Author	No. of Breast Cancers	RR	95% CI	P value
Persson[97]	634	.5	.4 - .6	—
Gambrell[98]	256	.53	—	<.007
Hunt[99]	50	.55	.28 - .96	—
Henderson[100]	—	.81	—	>.05
Criqui[101]	42	.73*	.44 – 1.22	—
Ewertz[102]	1,684	1.07	.88 – 1.3	—
Willis[103]	1,469†	.84‡	.75 - .94	—
Colditz[104]	1,935	1.14δ / .8‖	.85 – 1.51 / .6 – 1.07	—

* cancer mortality; †breast cancer deaths; ‡all cause mortality; δcurrent users; ‖prior users

These findings of apparently protective effects may arise from confounding factors, including the possibility that HRT may promote development of estrogen-dependent breast cancers that wither upon estrogen withdrawal. Another hypothesis is that HRT may stimulate growth of existing cancers, bringing them to light sooner. Nevertheless, the data are coherent in that they suggest that women who have used HRT and who develop breast cancer are not at increased risk of dying from breast cancer. Indeed, they may have a better prognosis than women who have never used HRT.

Reactivation of dormant tumor cells: The overriding concern among breast cancer survivors considering HRT is that it might hasten their demise. Although limited, there are reports of stimulation of breast cancer in women given hormones. A significant increase has been reported in the incorporation of tritiated thymidine in skin metastases among women treated with "physiological doses" of intramuscular estradiol and progesterone.[105]

Fabian et al. Used suppositories to obtain elevated serum levels of estradiol in women with stage IIIB breast cancer. Biopsies before and after HRT revealed that ER-positive breast cancers had a significant increase in S-phase fraction and proliferative index.[106] HRT withdrawal resulted in regression of metastatic breast cancer in four women.[107] Two cases of primary tumor regression after discontinuation of HRT have been described.[108,109] Alternative interpretations of these results have been presented.[110]

CONCLUSIONS

Ultimately, the question of how HRT affects mortality from all causes among breast cancer survivors can only be answered by a prospective, randomized trial requiring thousands of women. Many questions exist, and it is premature to mount such a trial without pilot data. Will oncologists accept such trials? Will breast cancer survivors be willing to participate in randomized trials of HRT? What are the baseline quality-of-life measurements in these women? How are they affected by HRT, especially among tamoxifen users? What is the proper dose of HRT in tamoxifen users? These questions and many others should be answered before larger trials are planned.

The beneficial effects of HRT on quality of life are indisputable. The impact on overall health is favorable as well. Theoretical concern over activating dormant tumor cells is not supported by existing clinical evidence.[111] Oncologists and their patients need more research like the prospective clinical trial of HRT in breast cancer survivors being conducted by Sellin et al. The primary endpoint of that trial is osteoporosis prevention. Another trial is being conducted by the Eastern Cooperative Oncology Group and will be open to women who have vasomotor or vaginal symptoms and are taking tamoxifen. They will be randomly assigned to receive HRT or placebo. Primary endpoints include accrual rate and symptom relief. The Southwest Oncology Group will study the effects of megestrol acetate at two doses and compare them with those of placebo in women with vasomotor symptoms. These clinical trials and others that are planned in Canada and Europe will provide valuable pilot information for the design of larger phase III studies.

ACKNOWLEDGEMENTS

The author gratefully acknowledges Ms. Joan David for editorial assistance.

REFERENCES

1.   Fisher B, Costantino J, Redmond C, et al. A randomized clinical trial evaluating tamoxifen in the treatment of patients with node-negative breast cancer who have estrogen-receptor-positive tumors. N Engl J Med 1989; 320:479.

2.   Poehlman ET, Toth MJ, Gardner AW. Changes in energy balance and body composition at menopause: A controlled longitudinal study. Ann Intern Med 1995; 123:673.

3.   The Writing Group for the PEPI Trial. Effects of estrogen/progestin regimens on heart disease risk factors in postmenopausal women: the Postmenopausal Estrogen/Progestin Interventions (PEPI) Trial. JAMA 1997; 278:1402.

4.   Huang Z, Hankinson SE, Colditz GA, et al. Dual effects of weight gain on breast cancer risk. JAMA 1997; 278:1407

5.   Sporrong T, Hellgran M, Samsioe G, Mattson LA. Comparison of four continuously administered progestogen plus oestradiol combinations for climacteric complaints. Br J Obstet Gynecol 1998; 95:1042

6.   Couzi RJ, Helzlsouer KJ, Fetting JH. Prevalence of menopausal symptoms among women with a history of breast cancer and attitudes toward estrogen replacement therapy. J Clin Oncol 1995; 13:2737

7.   Boulet MJ, Oddens BJ, Lehert P, Vemer HM, Viser A. Climacteric and menopause in seven south-east Asian countries. Maturitas 1994; 19:157.

8.   Loprinzi CL, Pisansky TM, Fonseca R, et al. Pilot evaluation of venlaxafine hydrochloride for the therapy of hot flashes in cancer survivors. J Clin Oncol 1998; 16:2377.

9.   Longacre TA, Bartow SA. A correlative morphologic study of human breast and endometrium in the menstrual cycle. Am J Surg Pathol 1986; 10:382.

10.   Potten CS, Watson RJ, Williams GT, Tickle S, Roberts SA, Harris M, Howell A. The effect of age and the menstrual cycle on the proliferative activity of the normal human breast. Br J Cancer 1988; 58:163.

11.   Anderson TJ, Battersby S, King RJB, McPherson K, Going JJ. Oral contraceptive use influences resting breast proliferation. Hum Pathol 1989; 20:1139

12.   Bergvist L, Adami Ho, Person I, et al. Prognosis after breast cancer diagnosis in women exposed to estrogen and estrogen-progestogen replacement therapy. Am J Epidemiol 1992; 130:221

13.   Huggins C, Yang NC. Induction and extinction of mammary cancer. Science 1962; 137:257.

14.   Diamond JE, Hollander VP. Progesterone and breast cancer. Mt Sinai J Med 1979; 46:225.

15.   Jordan VC, MK, Langan-Fahey S. Suppression of mouse mammary tumorigenesis by long term tamoxifen therapy. J Natl Cancer Inst 1991; 83:492.

16.   Kordon E, Lanari C, Meiss R, Elizade P, Charreau E,   Pasqualini, CD. Hormone dependence of a mouse mammary tumor line induced in vivo by medroxyprogesterone acetate. Breast Cancer Res Treat 1990; 33.

17.   Hissom JR, Moore MR. Progestin effects on growth in the human breast cancer cell lineT47D. Possible therapeutic implications. Biochem Biophys Res Commun 1987; 45:706

18.   Braunsburg H, Coldham NG, Wong W. Hormonal therapies for breast cancer: can progestogens stimulate growth? Cancer Letters 1986; 30:213.

19.   Nesheim BI, Saetre T. Reduction of menopausal hot flashes by methyldopa. Eur J Clin Pharmacol 1981; 20:413.

20.   Bergmans MGM, Merkus JM, Corbey RS, Schellekens LA, Ubachs JM. Effects of bellergal retard on climacteric complaints: a double-blind, placebo-controlled study. Maturitas 1987; 9:227.

21.   Lebherz TB, French L. Nonhormonal treatment of the menopausal syndrome. Obstet Gynecol 1969; 33:795.

22.   Goldberg RM, Loprinzi CL, O'Fallon JR, et al. Transdermal clonidine for ameliorating tamoxifen-induced hot flashes. J Clin Oncol 1994; 12:155.

23. Barton DL, Loprinzi CL, Quella SK, et al. Prospective evaluation of vitamin E for hot flashes in breast cancer survivors. J Clin Oncol 1998; 16:495.

24. Hirata JD, Swiersz LM, Zell B, Small R, Ettinger B. Does dong quai have estrogenic effects on postmenopausal women? A double-blind, placebo-controlled trial. Fertil Steril 1997; 68:981.

25. Loprinzi CL, Michalak JC, Quella SK, et al. Megestrol acetate for the prevention of hot flashes. N Engl J Med 1994; 331:347.

26. Morrison JC, Martin DC, Blair RA, et al. The use of medroxyprogesterone acetate for relief of climacteric symptoms. Am J Obstet Gynecol 1980; 138:99.

27. Albrecht BG, Schiff I, Tulchinsky D, Ryan KJ. Objective evidence that placebo and oral medroxyprogesterone acetate therapy diminish menopausal vasomotor flushes. Am J Obstet Gynecol 1981; 139:631.

28. Schiff I, Tuschinsky D, Cramer D. Oral medroxyprogesterone acetate in the treatment of postmenopausal symptoms. JAMA 1980; 224:1443.

29. Bullock JL, Massey FM, Cambrell RD Jr. Use of medroxyprogesterone acetae to prevent menopausal symptoms. Obstet Gynecol 1975; 46:165.

30. Mouridsen HT, Elleman K, Mattson W. Therapeutic effect of tamoxifen vs. tamoxifen combined with medroxyprogesterone acetate in advanced breast cancer in postmenopausal women. Cancer Treat Rep 1979; 63:171.

31. Gibson DFC, Johnson DA, Langan-Fahey SM, Lababidi MK, Wolberg WH, Jordan VC. The effects of intermittent progesterone upon tamoxifen inhibition of tumor growth in the 7, 12 dimethylbenzanthracene rat mammary tumor model. Breast Cancer Res Treat 1993; 27:283.

32. Delmas PD, Bjarnason NH, Mitlak BH, et al. Effects of raloxifene on bone mineral density, serum cholesterol concentrations, and uterine endometrium in postmenopausal women. N Engl J Med 1987; 337:1641.

33. Fisher B, Constantino JP, Wickerham DL, et al. Tamoxifen for prevention of breast cancer: report of the national surgical adjuvant breast and bowel project P-1 study. J Natl Cancer Inst 1998; 90:1371.

34. Powles TJ, Hickish T, Casey S, O'Brien M. Hormone replacement after breast cancer. Lancet 1993; 342:60.

35. Chang J, Powles TJ, Ashley SE, et al. The effect of tamoxifen and hormone replacement therapy on serum cholesterol, bone mineral density and coagulation factors in healthy postmenopausal women participating in a randomized, controlled tamoxifen prevention study. Ann Oncol 1996; 7:671.

36. Veronesi U, Maisonneux P, Costa A, et al. Prevention of breast cancer with tamoxifen: preliminary findings from the Italian randomized trial among hysterectomized women. Lancet 1998; 352:93.

37. Jones G, Nguyen T, Sambrook PN, Kelly PJ, Gilbert C,   Eisman JA. Symptomatic fracture incidence in elderly men and women: the Dubbo Osteoporosis Epidemiologic Study (DOES). Osteoporisis Int 1994; 2:277.

38. Saarto T, Blomqvist C, Valimaki M, Makela P, Sarna S,   Elomaa I. Chemical castration induced by adjuvant cyclophosphamide, methotrexate, and fluorouracil chemotherapy causes rapid bone loss that is reduced by clodronate: a randomized study in premenopausal breast cancer patients. J Clin Oncol 1997; 15:1341.

39. Prince RL. Diet and the prevention of osteoporotic fractures. N Engl J Med 1997; 336:701.

40. The writing group for the PEPI trial. Effects of hormone therapy on bone mineral density. JAMA 1996; 276:1389.

41. Love RR, Mazess RB, Barden HS, et al. Effects of tamoxifen on bone mineral density in postmenopausal women with breast cancer. N Engl J Med 1992; 326:852.

42. Delmas PD, Bjarnason NH, Mitlak BH, et al. Effects of raloxifene on bone mineral density, serum cholesterol concentrations, and uterine endometrium in postmenopausal women. N Engl J Med 1998; 337:1641

43. McClung M, Clemmesen B, Daifotis A, et al. Alendronate prevents postmenopausal bone loss in women without osteoporosis. Ann Intern Med.1998; 128:253.

44. Hosking D, Chilvers CE, Christiansen C, et al. Prevention of bone loss with alendronate in postmenopausal women under 60 years of age. N Engl J Med 1998; 338:485.

45. Grady D , Rubin SM, Petitti DB, et al. Hormone therapy to prevent disease and prolong life in postmenopausal women. Ann Intern Med 1992; 15:1016.

46. Kiel DP, Felson DT, Anderson JJ, et al. Hip fracture and the use of estrogens in postmenopausal women. N Engl J Med 1987; 317:1169.

47. Liberman UA, Weiss SR, Broll J, et al. Effect of oral alendronate on bone mineral density and the incidence of fractures in postmenopausal osteoporosis. N Engl J Med 1995; 333: 1437.

48. Stampfer MJ, Hennekens CH, Manson JE, Colditz GA, Rosner B, Willett WC. Vitamin E consumption and the risk of coronary disease in women. N Engl J Med 1993; 328:1444.

49. Rimm EB, Willett WC, Hu FB, et al. Folate and vitamin B_6 from diet and supplements in relation to the risk of coronary heart disease among women. JAMA 1998; 279:359.

50. Bines J, Oleske DM, Cobleigh MA. Ovarian function in premenopausal women treated with adjuvant chemotherapy for breast cancer. J Clin Oncol 1996; 14:1718.

51. Mansour EG, Gray R, Shatila AH, et al. Efficacy of adjuvant chemotherapy in high-risk node-negative breast cancer. N Engl J Med 1989; 320:485

52. The Ludwig Breast Cancer Study Group. Prolonged disease-free survival after one course of perioperative adjuvant chemotherapy for node-negative breast cancer. N Engl J Med 1989; 320:491.

53. Fisher B, Redmond C, Dimitrov NV, et al. A randomized trial evaluating sequential methotrexate and fluorouracil in the treatment of patients with node-negative breast cancer who have estrogen-receptor negative tumors. N Engl J Med 1989; 320:474.

54. Barrett-Connor E, Bush TL. Estrogen and coronary disease in women. Clinical Cardiology JAMA 1991; 265:1861.

55. Stampfer MJ, Colditz GA, Willett WC, et al. Postmenopausal estrogen therapy and cardiovascular disease. Ten-year follow-up from the nurses' health study. N Engl J Med 1991; 325:756.

56. Rosen PP, Groshen S, Kinne DW, et al. Factors influencing prognosis in node negative breast carcinoma: Analysis of 767 T1N0M0/T2N0M0 patients with long-term followup. J Clin Oncol 1993; 11:2090.

57. Early Breast Cancer Trialists' Collaborative Group. Polychemotherapy for early breast cancer: An overview of the randomized trials. Lancet 1998; 352:930.

58. Fisher B, Dignam J, Wolmark N, et al. Tamoxifen and chemotherapy for lymph node-negative, estrogen receptor-positive breast cancer. J Natl Cancer Inst 1997; 89:1673.

59. Antiplatelet Trialists' Collaboration. Collaborative overview of randomized trials of antiplatelet therapy-I: Prevention of death, myocardial infarction and stroke by prolonged antiplatelet therapy in various categories of patients. Br Med J 1994; 308:81.

60. Scandinavian Simvastatin Survival Study Group. Randomized trial of cholesterol lowering in 4444 patients with coronary heart disease: the Scandinavian Simvastatin Survival Study (4S). Lancet 1994; 344:1383.

61. Downs JR, Clearfield M, Weis S, Whitney E, Shapiro DR, Beere PA, et al. Primary prevention of acute coronary events with Lovastatin in men and women with average cholesterol levels. JAMA 1998; 279:1615.

62. Barrett-Connor E, Bush TL, Estrogen and coronary heart disease in women. Clinical Cardiology JAMA 1991; 265:1861.

63. Lobo RA. Cardiovascular implications of estrogen replacement therapy. Obstet Gynecol 1990; 75(Suppl4): 18S25S.

64. Walsh BW, Kuller, LH, Wild RA, et al. Effects of raloxifene on serum lipids and coagulation factors in healthy postmenopausal women. JAMA 1988; 279:1445.

65. Early Breast Cancer Trialists' Collaborative Group. Tamoxifen for early breast cancer: an overview of the randomized trials. Lancet 1998; 351:1451.

66. Clarkson TB, Cline JM, Williams JK, Anthony MS. Gonadal hormone substitutes: effects on the cardiovascular system. Osteoporosis Int 1997; Suppl I:S43.

67. Saarto T, Blomqvist C, Ehnholm C, Taskinen RM, Elomaa I. Antiatherogenic effects of adjuvant antiestrogens: a randomized trial comparing the effects of tamoxifen and toremifene on plasma lipid levels in postmenopausal women with node-positive breast cancer. J Clin Oncol 1996; 14:429.

68. Anderson JW, Johnstone B, Cook-Newell ME, Meta-analysis of the effects of soy protein intake on serum lipids. N Engl J Med 1995; 333:276.

69. Decensi A, Bonanni B, Guerriieri-Gonzaga A, et al. Biologic activity of tamoxifen at low doses in healthy women. J Natl Cancer Inst 1998; 90:1461.

70. Anthony MS, Clarkson TB, Hughes CI Jr, Morgan TM, Burke GL. Soybean isoflavones improve cardiovascular risk factors without affecting the reproductive system of peripubertal rhesus monkeys. J Nutr 1996; 126:43.

71. Yaffe K, Sawaya G, Lieberburg I, Grady D. Estrogen therapy in postmenopausal women: effects on cognitive function and dementia. JAMA 1998; 279:688.

72. Schiff I, Wentworth B, KoosB, Tulchinsky D, Ryan KJ. Effect of estradiol administration on the hypogonadal woman. Fertil Steril 1978; 30:278.

73. Mattson LA, Cullberg G. Vaginal absorption of two estradiol preparations. Acta Obstet Gynecol Scand 1983; 62:393.

74. Heimer GM. Estradiol in the menopause. Acta Obstet Gynecol Scand 1987; Suppl 139:23P.
75. Handa VL, Bachus Ke, Johnston WE, Robboy SJ, Hammond CB. Vaginal administration of low-dose conjugated estrogens: systemic absorption and effects on the endometrium. Obstet Gynecol 1994; 84:215.
76. Smith P, Heimer G, Lindskog M, Ulmsten A. Oestradiol-releasing vaginal ring for treatment of postmenopausal urogenital atrophy. Maturitas 16:145-154, 1993.
77. Nachtigall LE. Comparative study: Replens versus local estrogen in menopausal women. Fertil Steril 61:178, 1994.
78. Loprinzi CL, Abu-Ghazaleh Sloan JA, et al. Phase III randomized double-blind study to evaluate the efficacy of a polycarbophil-based vaginal moisturizer in women with breast cancer. J Clin Oncol 15:969, 1997.
79. Cable E, Miracle-McMahill H, Than MJ and Heath C. Estrogen replacement therapy and risk of fatal colon cancer in a prospective cohort of postmenopausal women. J Natl Cancer Inst 87:517, 1995.
80. Grodstein F, Martinez ME, Platz EA, et al. Postmenopausal hormone use and risk for colorectal cancer and adenoma. Ann Intern Med 128:705, 1998.
81. Potter JK, Bostick RM, Grandits GA, et al. Hormone replacement therapy is associated with lower risk of adenomatous polyps of the large bowel: the Minnesota Cancer Prevention research unit case-control study. Cancer Epidemiology, Biomarkers and Prevention 5:779, 1996.
82. Cline JM, Soderqvist G, von Schoultz E, Skoog L, von Schoultz B. Effects of hormone replacement therapy on the mammary gland of surgically postmenopausal cynomolgus macaques. Am J Obstet Gynecol 174:93, 1996.
83. Laya MB, Gallagher JC, Schreiman JS, et al. Effect of postmenopausal hormonal replacement therapy on mammographic density and parenchymal pattern. Radiology 196:433, 1995.
84. McNicholas MMJ, Geneghan JP, Milner MH, et al. Pain and increased mammographic density in women receiving hormone replacement therapy: a prospective study. AJR 163:311, 1994.
85. Persson I, Thurfjell E, Holmberg L. Effect of estrogen and estrogen-progestin replacement regimens on mammographic breast parenchymal density. J. Clin Oncol 15:3201, 1997.
86. Kelsey JL, Berkowitz GS. Breast cancer epidemiology. Cancer Res 48:5615, 1988.

87. Harvey EB, Brinton LA. Second cancer following cancer of the breast in Connecticut, 1935-1982. In: Boice JD Jr, Storm HH, Curtis RE, eds. Multiple primary cancers in Connecticut and Denmark. National Cancer Institute monograph 68. Washington, D.C.: Government Printing Office, 99-112, 1985 (NIH publication no. 85-2714).

88. Henrich JB. The postmenopausal estrogen/breast cancer controversy. JAMA 268:1900, 1992.

89. DuPont WD, Page DL. Menopausal estrogen replacement therapy and breast cancer. Arch Intern Med 151:67, 1991.

90. Steinberg KK, Thacker SB, Smith SJ, et al. A meta-analysis of the effect of estrogen replacement therapy on the risk of breast cancer. JAMA 265:1985, 1991.

91. Armstrong BK. Oestrogen therapy after the menopause – boon or bane? Med J Aust 248:113, 1988.

92. Grady D, Ernster V. Invited commentary: Does postmenopausal hormone therapy cause breast cancer? Am J Epidemiol 134:1396, 1991.

93. Sillero-Arenas M, Delgado-Rodriguez M, Rodrigues-Canteras R, et al. Menopausal hormone replacement therapy and breast cancer: a meta-analysis. Obstet Gynecol 79:286, 1992.

94. Colditz GA, Egan KM, Stampfer MJ. Hormone replacement therapy and risk of breast cancer: results from epidemiologic studies. Am J Obstet Gynecol 168:1473, 1993.

95. Ginsburg ES, Mello NK, Mendelson JK, et al. Effects of alcohol ingestion on estrogens in postmenopausal women. JAMA 276:1747, 1996.

96. Nayfield SG, Karp JE, Ford LG, et al. Potential role of tamoxifen in prevention of breast cancer. J Natl Cancer Inst 83:1450, 1991.

97. Persson I, Yuen J, Gergkvist L, Schairer C. Cancer incidence and mortality in women receiving estrogen and estrogen-progestin replacement therapy – long-term follow-up of a Swedish cohort. Int J Cancer 67:327, 1996.

98. Gambrell DR. Proposal to decrease the risk and improve the prognosis in breast cancer. Am J Obstet Gynecol 150:119, 1984.

99. Hunt K, Vessey M, McPherson K, Coleman M. Long-term surveillance of mortality and cancer incidence in women receiving hormone replacement therapy. Br J Obstet Gynecol 94:620, 1987.

100. Henderson BE, Paganini-Hill A, Ross RK. Decreased mortality in users of estrogen replacement therapy. Arch Intern Med 151:75, 1991.

101. Criqui MH, Suarez L, Barrett-Connor E, et al. Postmenopausal estrogen use and mortality. Am J Epidemiol 128:606, 1988.

102. Ewertz M, Gillanders S, Meyer L, Zedeler K. Survival of breast cancer patients in relation to factors which affect the risk of developing breast cancer. Int J Cancer 49:526, 1991.

103. Wilis DB, Calle EE, Miracle-McMahill HL, Heath Jr CW. Cancer Causes and Control. 7:449-457, 1996.

104. Colditz GA, Hankinson SE, Hunter DJ, et al. The use of estrogens and progestins and the risk of breast cancer in postmenopausal women. N Engl J Med 332:1589, 1995.

105. Dao TL, Sinha DI, Nemoto T, Patel J. Effect of estrogen and progesterone on cellular replication of human breast tumors. Cancer Res 42:359, 1982.

106. Fabian CJ, Kimler BF, McKittrick R, et al. Recruitment with high physiological doses of estradiol preceding chemotherapy: flow cytometric and therapeutic results in women with locally advanced breast cancer – a Southwest Oncology Group Study. Cancer Res 54:5357, 1994.

107. Dhodapkar MV, Ingle NJ, Ahmann DL. Estrogen replacement therapy withdrawal and regression of metastatic breast cancer. Cancer 75:43, 1995.

108. Powles TJ, Hickish T. Breast cancer response to hormone replacement therapy withdrawal. Lancet 345:1442, 1995.

109. Harvey SC, DiPiro PJ, Meyer JE. Marked regression of a nonpalpable breast cancer after cessation of hormone replacement therapy. AJR 167:394, 1996.

110. Cobleigh MA. Hormone replacement therapy in breast cancer survivors. In: Diseases of the Breast Updates. Harris JR, Lippman ME, eds. 1:1, 1997.

111. Eden JA, Bush T, Nand S, Wren BG. The Royal Hospital for Women Breast Cancer Study: a case-controlled study of combined continuous hormone replacement therapy amongst women with a personal history of breast cancer. Menopause 2:67, 1995.

2

Sentinel Lymphadenectomy In Node Negative Breast Cancer

Philip I. Haigh, M.D., FRCS(C)
Clinical Fellow, Surgical Oncology
John Wayne Cancer Institute

Armando E. Giuliano, M.D.
Chief of Surgical Oncology
John Wayne Cancer Institute at Saint John's Health Center
Clinical Professor of Surgery
UCLA School of Medicine

From the Joyce Eisenberg Keefer Breast Center, and the Division of Surgical Oncology, John Wayne Cancer Institute at Saint John's Health Center, Santa Monica, CA.

Supported in part by funding from the Ben B. and Joyce E. Eisenberg Foundation, Los Angeles, California, and the Fashion Footwear Association of New York.

INTRODUCTION

Axillary lymphadenectomy (ALND) remains the gold standard for identifying axillary nodal metastases and managing patients with early stage breast cancer.[1] A level I and II ALND accurately stages the patient, allowing for prognostication and decisions regarding adjuvant therapy. Furthermore, excellent regional control is achieved with ALND, with subsequent axillary recurrence a rare event.[2,3] There may be an improvement in survival after ALND, however, this remains debatable. As the use of screening mammography increases, the size of primary breast cancers has been progressively diminishing over the last few decades, concomitant with a declining proportion of patients who have axillary metastases.[4]

ALND may have substantial associated morbidity. Occasionally, injury to major vessels or motor nerves may occur. Significant lymphedema after ALND may occur early or years later, with an incidence as high as 30% in some series.[5-7] With data supporting adjuvant chemotherapy regardless of nodal status,[8,9] routine ALND for all patients with early breast cancer is being questioned.[4,10,11] For these reasons, sentinel lymphadenectomy (SLND) was developed in breast cancer using a vital dye to identify the sentinel node, the lymph node most likely to harbor metastases if they are present. Those patients with nodal metastases may be identified who may derive a benefit from ALND, and also have the highest potential benefit from adjuvant therapy. More importantly, those patients whose sentinel nodes do not contain metastases may be spared ALND and avoid its associated morbidity. Thus, ALND may be reserved for those patients with identifiable lymph node metastases.

SLND USING BLUE DYE

Intraoperative lymphatic mapping and SLND was developed by Morton and colleagues for use in patients with melanoma.[12] The procedure successfully identified lymph nodes which accurately represented the status of the regional drainage basin. With some major modifications of their technique, mainly because of differences in kinetics of blue dye transit in breast tissue compared to skin, Giuliano et al. examined whether SLND could accurately predict the presence or absence of axillary metastases in patients with breast cancer. As an initial feasibility trial, SLND was performed using isosulfan vital blue dye (Lymphazurin®), which was followed by completion ALND in 174 consecutive procedures; nearly all patients were used to establish the optimal technique necessary to identify the sentinel node, varying such factors as dye volume and timing of dissection after injection.[13] Sentinel nodes were found in 114 of the 174 procedures (66%) and correctly predicted the remaining axillary nodes in 109 (96%) cases. After this development phase, in 107 SLND procedures that were followed by an ALND, one or more sentinel nodes were successfully identified in 94% of cases, and were 100% correct in predicting axillary status.[14]

In a parallel study, the results of routine pathologic evaluation of the ALND specimen in patients who had ALND only were compared to the results of multiple sectioning and immunohistochemistry (IHC) evaluation of the sentinel node in a separate group of patients who had SLND followed by complete ALND. IHC staining of multiple sections of the sentinel node significantly increased the accuracy and detection rate of metastases when compared to routine histopathologic processing of the ALND specimen.[15] Scrutiny of one or two sentinel nodes improved the detection of axillary metastases when compared to examination of hematoxylin and eosin (H&E) sections from all nodes in the ALND specimen.

The assumption that the status of the sentinel node will predict the status of the entire axilla was recently validated. Histopathologic examination of sentinel nodes previously used both H&E and IHC, and the non-sentinel nodes in the axillary specimen were processed with H&E only. In 60 patients whose sentinel nodes were negative for metastases by IHC and H&E, 1,087 non-sentinel nodes were also examined using both IHC and H&E on multiple sections. No metastases were found in the non-sentinel nodes by H&E, but only one of these nodes converted to tumor-positive by IHC.[16] This strongly supports the hypothesis that if the sentinel node is tumor free, then non-sentinel nodes will be tumor free.

SLND USING RADIOPHARMACEUTICALS

Other groups have successfully adopted SLND also using blue dye.[18-21] However, other methods of SLND also support the sentinel node concept. Radiopharmaceuticals can be used as the mapping agent, which travel to the sentinel node after injection at the primary site. Radioactive sentinel nodes are then identified intraoperatively using a hand-held gamma probe, a technique first described by Krag.[22] Depending on the agent used, the radiocolloid is injected one hour prior or up to 24 hours before the procedure. Common radiopharmaceuticals in use are technetium-99m-labeled sulfur colloid, human albumin colloid or antimony, which may be injected peritumorally or subdermally, and radioactive sentinel nodes are removed until the surrounding counts normalize to background levels.[23-30] Veronesi and colleagues reported on

163 patients who underwent SLND using technetium- labeled human albumin colloid particles.[23] They injected radioisotope subdermally superficial to the tumor to map the sentinel node using a gamma probe. In 98% of patients the sentinel node was identified and correctly predicted the axillary status in 97% of patients. A large multicenter trial of SLND has corroborated the validity of the sentinel node concept.[25] This trial, using radiocolloid and intraoperative gamma probe detection as the mapping technique, reported that the sentinel node was 97% accurate in predicting the status of the axillary nodes. Sentinel nodes were identified in 91% of cases. The rate of sentinel node identification varied significantly among the 11 experienced breast surgeons participating in the trial. The overall false negative rate of 11.4% was concerning since the surgeons in the study who enrolled more than 40 patients had a false-negative rate of between 6.3% and 28.6%, which was not statistically significant. Each surgeon had to perform 5 proctored procedures before entering patients into the trial: clearly, the technique of SLND with radioisotope requires appropriate training to acquire the expertise necessary to achieve dependable SLND results.

Some investigators have combined the two approaches by using both blue dye and radiocolloid to achieve excellent results.[17,31-34] The study by Albertini and colleagues utilized Lymphazurin® dye and filtered technetium sulfur-colloid as lymphatic mapping agents.[31] The sentinel node identification rate was 92%, the majority found by both blue dye and radiocolloid. Eighteen sentinel nodes contained metastases, all of which were identified by both dye and colloid. Albertini *et al.* concluded that the combination of dye and colloid increased sentinel node identification and is therefore superior to radiocolloid or dye alone.

Table 1 summarizes the results of the three general techniques used for SLND in breast cancer. The accuracy of the three techniques is similar. Radiocolloid for lesions in the upper outer quadrant may be inferior to blue dye for sentinel node identification, because "shine through" from the primary injection site can interfere with sentinel node identification the two are in close proximity. This probably contributed to the majority of false negative results in the multicenter trial by Krag, all which occurred with tumors in the lateral half of the breast.[25] On the other hand, a sentinel node that maps outside the axilla will not be identified using blue dye, whereas radioguided surgery will identify drainage to non-axillary sites. There is limited information on SLND for these non-axillary sites; although these sites have been documented, rarely have clinical metastases in early breast cancer been seen outside the axilla.[25] Internal mammary node SLND needs further study. Only in rare cases is there isolated drainage to the internal mammary nodes without axillary drainage, and so using blue dye alone should succeed in the vast majority of cases. We now obtain lymphoscintigrams for lesions in the medial breast prior to blue dye SLND because of the increased propensity for medial lesions to drain to internal mammary nodes in addition to the axilla; this allows correlation of successful sentinel node detection with the drainage pattern outlined by the lymphoscintigram.

CANDIDATE SELECTION FOR SLND

Most patients clinically node-negative breast carcinoma can undergo SLND. Care should be taken in patients with tumors larger than 6 cm or with a large excisional biopsy cavities, but SLND is feasible for these patients. Patients with multicentric tumors are not ideal candidates, but this is a relative contraindication requiring further investigation; multifocal tumors within the same quadrant could undergo SLND. Patients with high-grade DCIS continue to be entered into our experimental protocols, but SLND should not be done for DCIS because of the low, if any, incidence of metastases. A recent series detected sentinel node metastases in 4.6% of patients with DCIS[17], a significantly higher incidence than the historical rate of about 1%. This finding may indicate that not all breast cancer cells in lymph nodes are clinically significant metastases. It has been shown that vacuum-assisted biopsy of DCIS can dislodge epithelium into the stroma, which may mimic invasion; whether this displaced epithelium can gain entry into the lymphatics and lodge in the sentinel node has not been proven.[35]

OPERATIVE TECHNICAL DETAILS

After induction of general anesthesia or deep IV sedation, the patient is prepared and draped with the arm free to allow for its movement. The procedure begins with injection of 1% isosulfan blue dye (Lymphazurin®) around the tumor into the breast parenchyma on the axillary side of the tumor. Elevating the breast prevents subfascial or intrapectoral injection. For those cancers diagnosed with excisional biopsy, injection should be into the wall of the biopsy cavity and surrounding tissue; dye will not translocate into the lymphatics if injected into a seroma-filled biopsy cavity. If a lumpectomy is being performed for a non-palpable carcinoma, then the dye injection is made at the tip of the localizing wire, or through the localizing needle.

     Up to 5 cc of dye is used, with less volume, about 3 cc, for lesions closer to the axilla. Less volume is important for lesions high in the upper-outer quadrant, because blue dye may flood the axilla, making identification of the blue node particularly difficult. After injection, gentle massage of the breast enhances lymphatic uptake of dye.

SLND is delayed after dye injection depending on the location of the primary lesion. For lesions in the axillary tail, dissection should start about three minutes after injection, whereas lesions in the lower inner quadrant require about seven to ten minutes for adequate dye transit to the sentinel node. For the other areas of the breast, a five minute delay suffices. Timing of SLND is crucial, for a blue-stained sentinel node may lose its color intensity if too long a delay, or the blue dye may have not reached the sentinel node if performed too early.

A small transverse incision is made about 1 cm inferior to the hair-bearing area of the axillary skin. Subcutaneous tissue is incised with electrocautery, and dissection proceeds perpendicular to the skin to the clavi-pectoral fascia. Superficial, subcutaneous blue lymphatics can be transected; these should not be confused with lymphatics that drain to the sentinel node and are located deep to the clavi-pectoral fascia. The clavi-pectoral fascia is incised to search for a blue lymphatic channel, which is followed both superiorly and inferiorly. Abducting and flexing the arm helps to bring the axillary contents closer to the incision. Fine forceps are can be used to trace the blue lymphatic to a blue lymph node, representing the sentinel node. The sentinel node will either stain entirely or partially blue. Often just a small portion of its hilum near the afferent lymphatic will be blue. It is critical not to disrupt the delicate blue lymphatic channel, or identification of the sentinel node will be more difficult. Any bleeding must be controlled promptly, as blood will obscure the blue sentinel node. After removing the sentinel node, the afferent blue lymphatic must be followed proximally towards the breast to ensure no more proximal blue nodes are present.

Wide variations in technique exist when SLND is performed using radiopharmaceuticals. The specific radiopharmaceutical used, colloid particle size, timing of injection, method and volume of injection, and detection techniques all differ among series. The radioisotope most commonly used is technetium-99m, a high-energy radioisotope that decays by pure gamma emission. With a short half-life of 6 hours, technetium-99m is ideal for detection of a sentinel node with a gamma camera or probe. Colloidal radiopharmaceuticals labeled with technetium-99m are most commonly used for SLND. Antimony sulfide colloid (5-30 nm), or nanocolloid, a human albumin colloid usually less than 80 nm, are small particles only available commercially outside the United States.[36] Sulfur colloid, the most commonly employed agent in the United States, contains particles that range from 100-1000 nm. Debate continues regarding particle size; nevertheless, excellent results are achieved with either filtered sulfur colloid containing particles less than 200 nm, or with the unfiltered preparation which contains larger particles.[22,25] Injection of radiocolloid can be performed on the same day of surgery, or up to 24 hours prior to operation. Some investigators use preoperative lymphoscintigraphy,[26,30] while others use solely a hand-held gamma probe intraoperatively.[25] The optimal approach using radiopharmaceuticals has not yet been established, although the success in identifying the sentinel node using these variations in technique has been similar.

Infiltration of radiopharmaceutical is most often performed around the tumor or excision cavity in divided volumes, but a subdermal injection using smaller volumes has also been described.[23,30] Lymphoscintigraphy or a gamma probe can identify the hot spot over the skin, which should be marked with ink. SLND is then performed using the same technique as with the blue dye, starting with a skin incision over the hot spot, but in this case using the gamma probe covered with a sterile sheath to assist with sentinel node localization. Sentinel nodes are removed until counts return to background levels. Lesions in the high upper outer quadrant may require resection of the injection site before SLND to allow the gamma probe to distinguish radioactive sentinel nodes from surrounding radioactivity at the primary site.

After SLND, standard lumpectomy or total mastectomy is performed. The axillary wound after SLND is irrigated and closed without drainage. ALND is performed if the sentinel node contains any detectable tumor cells. In some centers, if the sentinel lymph node is free of metastases, ALND is not performed, which should be part of an experimental protocol. Recurrences have yet to be reported in patients who have SLND only for a sentinel node free of metastases.

HISTOPATHOLOGIC EXAMINATION OF SENTINEL NODE

The excised sentinel nodes are bisected and usually examined intraoperatively by frozen section of one or two levels using Diff-Quik. Paraffin sections are evaluated by hematoxylin and eosin staining (H&E) of 3-4 step sections, and if negative, immunohistochemistry (IHC) of the sections is performed using anti-cytokeratin antibodies. If frozen section is not done, deeper or additional sections may be examined by H&E and IHC. A small amount of tissue may be saved for molecular studies.

COMPLICATIONS OF SLND

Local complications after SLND are rare. No injuries to the long thoracic, thoracodorsal, or intercostobrachial nerves have been reported. The incidence of lymphedema is unknown, but will probably be low, equivalent to that for excisional lymph node biopsy. Side effects from isosulfan blue are also infrequent. The skin overlying the injection site may turn an obvious blue color. This will usually disappear over several days or weeks, but occasionally a slight bluish hue will persist in the breast for months, which is usually not bothersome for the patient. Local adverse effects from radiocolloid are uncommon, but patients occasionally complain of burning at the injection site. Furthermore, the breast can receive significant radiation doses with infiltration of radiocolloid, but usually resection of the area follows injection, obviating prolonged radiation exposure in the local tissues.[37] Systemic problems rarely arise from the use of blue dye. Absorption of isosulfan blue soon after injection can spuriously lower the capillary hemoglobin saturation as measured by pulse oximetry. This occurs because isosulphan blue has a peak wavelength of absorption similar to desoxyhemoglobin.[38] Patients should be warned that because some of the dye is excreted by the kidney, the urine may be green for 12-24 hours. Also, since the majority of drug is excreted into the bile, some patients may note blue-colored stools. Rare minor allergic reactions have been documented, as have a few major anaphylactic reactions after subcutaneous injection.[39] Mixing local anesthetic with the blue dye in the same syringe should not be done, because a solid precipitate will form, which may increase the risk for allergic reactions.[39] Minor and major allergic reactions have also been reported from radiocolloid. Overall, however, SLND is tolerated extremely well compared to ALND.

SUMMARY

SLND, regardless of method, can precisely predict the status of the axillary lymph nodes. Despite differences in technique, the consistent results support the sentinel node hypothesis in breast cancer. The procedure is well tolerated, and staging can be achieved accurately with minimal morbidity. SLND is a minimally-invasive procedure that provides tissue for the pathologist that represents the site most likely to harbor metastases. If a negative sentinel node is removed at SLND, it equates to truly node-negative breast cancer in almost all cases when done by experienced surgeons familiar with the technique.

SLND can be mastered by surgeons at several institutions, but requires appropriate training to learn the technique. The team involved in SLND, which consists of the surgeon, pathologist and nuclear medicine physician, must determine its own false negative rate for the procedure, which requires a concomitant ALND so that accuracy is validated. Multicenter randomized clinical trials from the American College of Surgeons and NSABP are in progress, which will evaluate in general, although with different randomization schemes, the outcome of patients who have SLND alone compared to those who have ALND. Before ALND is completely abandoned, these trials must be completed so that the role of SLND in the management of all patients with early breast cancer is fully defined.

REFERENCES

1. National Institutes of Health. NIH consensus conference on the treatment of early-stage breast cancer. JAMA 265:391-395, 1991.
2. Halverson KJ, Taylor ME, Perez CA, et al. Regional nodal management and patterns of failure following conservative surgery and radiation therapy for stage I and II breast cancer. Int J Radiat Oncol Biol Phys 26:593-599, 1993.
3. Recht A, Pierce SM, Abner A, et al. Regional node failure after conservative surgery and radiotherapy for early-stage breast carcinoma. J Clin Oncol 9:988-996, 1991.
4. Cady B, Stone MD, Schuler JG, et al. The new era in breast cancer: invasion, size, and nodal involvement dramatically decreasing as a result of mammographic screening. Arch Surg 131:301-308, 1996.
5. Keramopoulos A, Tsionou C, Minaretzis D, et al. Arm morbidity following treatment of breast cancer with total axillary dissection: A multivariated approach. Oncology 50:445-449, 1993.
6. Ivens D, Hoe AL, Podd TJ, et al. Assessment of morbidity from complete axillary dissection. Br J Cancer 66:136-138, 1992.
7. Larson D, Weinstein M, Goldberg I, et al. Edema of the arm as a function of the extent of axillary surgery in patients with stage I-II carcinoma of the breast treated with primary radiotherapy. Int J Radiat Oncol Biol Phys 12:1575-1582, 1986.
8. Early Breast Cancer Trialists' Collaborative Group. Systemic treatment of early breast cancer by hormonal, cytotoxic, or immune therapy. Lancet 339:1-15, 1992.

9. Early Breast Cancer Trialists' Collaborative Group. Systemic treatment of early breast cancer by hormonal, cytotoxic, or immune therapy. Lancet 339:71-85, 1992.

10. Silverstein MJ, Gierson ED, Waisman JR, et al. Axillary lymph node dissection for T1a breast carcinoma. Is it indicated? Cancer 73:664-667, 1994.

11. Jamali FR, Kurtzman SH, Deckers PJ. Role of axillary dissection in mammographically detected breast cancer. Surg Oncol Clin Nor Am 6:343-358, 1997.

12. Morton DL, Wen DR, Wong JH, et al. Technical details of intraoperative lymphatic mapping for early stage melanoma. Arch Surg 127:392-399, 1992.

13. Giuliano AE, Kirgan DM, Guenther JM, et al. Lymphatic mapping and sentinel lymphadenectomy for breast cancer. Ann Surg 220:391-401, 1994.

14. Giuliano AE, Jones RC, Brennan M, et al. Sentinel lymphadenectomy in breast cancer. J Clin Oncol 15:2345-2350, 1997.

15. Giuliano AE, Dale PS, Turner RR, et al. Improved axillary staging of breast cancer with sentinel lymphadenectomy. Ann Surg 222:394-401, 1995.

16. Turner RR, Ollila DW, Krasne DL, et al. Histopathological validation of the sentinel lymph node hypothesis for breast carcinoma. Ann Surg 226:271-278, 1997.

17. Cox CE, Pendas S, Cox JM, et al. Guidelines for sentinel node biopsy and lymphatic mapping of patients with breast cancer. Ann Surg 227:645-653, 1998.

18. Guenther JM, Krishnamoorthy M, Tan LR. Sentinel lymphadenectomy for breast cancer in a community managed care setting. Cancer J Sci Am 3:336-340, 1997.

19. Koller M, Barsuk D, Zippel D, et al. Sentinel lymph node involvement: a predictor for axillary node status with breast cancer – has the time come? Eur J Surg Oncol 24:166-168, 1998.

20. Flett MM, Going JJ, Stanton PD et al. Sentinel node localization in patients with breast cancer. Br J Surg 85:991-993, 1998.

21. Dale PS, Williams JT, IV. Axillary staging utilizing selective sentinel lymphadenectomy for patients with invasive breast carcinoma. Am Surg 64:28-32, 1998.

22. Krag DN, Weaver DL, Alex JC, et al. Surgical resection and radiolocalization of the sentinel lymph node in breast cancer using a gamma probe. Surg Oncol 2:335-339, 1993.

23. Veronesi U, Paganelli G, Galimberti V, et al. Sentinel-node biopsy to avoid axillary dissection in breast cancer with clinically negative lymph-nodes. Lancet 349:1864-1867, 1997.
24. Pijpers R, Meijer S, Hoekstra OS, et al. Impact of lymphoscintigraphy on sentinel node identification with Technetium-99m-colloidal albumin in breast cancer. J Nucl Med 38:366-368, 1997.
25. Krag D, Weaver D, Ashikaga T, et al. The sentinel node in breast cancer. NEJM 339:941-946, 1998.
26. Borgstein PJ, Pijpers R, Comans EF, et al. Sentinel lymph node biopsy in breast cancer: guidelines and pitfalls of lymphoscintigraphy and gamma probe detection. J Am Coll Surg 186:275-283, 1998.
27. Crossin JA, Johnson AC, Stewart PB, et al. Gamma-probe-guided resection of the sentinel lymph node in breast cancer. Am Surg 64:666-669, 1998.
28. Miner TJ, Shriver CD, Jaques DP, et al. Ultrasonographically guided injection improves localization of the radiolabeled sentinel lymph node in breast cancer. Ann Surg Oncol 5:315-321, 1998.
29. Offodile R, Hoh C, Barsky SH, et al. Minimally invasive breast carcinoma staging using lymphatic mapping with radiolabeled dextran. Cancer 82:1704-8, 1998.
30. De Cicco C, Cremonesi M, Luini A, et al. Lymphoscintigraphy and radioguided biopsy of the sentinel axillary node in breast cancer J Nucl Med 12:2080-4, 1998.
31. Albertini JJ, Lyman GH, Cox C, et al. Lymphatic mapping and sentinel node biopsy in the patient with breast cancer. JAMA 276:1818-1822, 1996.
32. Borgstein PJ, Meijer S, Pijpers R. Intradermal blue dye to identify sentinel lymphnode in breast cancer. Lancet 349:1668-1669, 1997.
33. O'Hea BJ, Hill ADK, El-Shirbiny AM, et al. Sentinel lymph node biopsy in breast cancer: initial experience at Memorial Sloan-Kettering Cancer Center. J Am Coll Surg 186:423-427, 1998.
34. Barnwell JM, Arredondo MA, Kollmorgen D, et al. Sentinel node biopsy in breast cancer. Ann Surg Oncol 5:126-130, 1998.
35. Liberman L, Vuolo M, Dershaw DD et al. Epithelial displacement after stereotactic 11-gauge directional vacuum-assisted breast biopsy. AJR 172:677-81, 1999.
36. Glass EC, Essner R, Giuliano AE. Sentinel node localization in breast cancer. Sem Nuc Med 24:57-68, 1999.
37. Glass EC, Basinski JE, Krasne DL, Giuliano AE. Radiation safety considerations for sentinel node techniques. Ann Surg Oncol 6:10-1, 1999.

38. Larsen VH, Freundendal-Pedersen A, Fogh-Andersen N. The influence of Patent Blue V on pulse oximetry and haemoximetry. Acta Anaes Scand 39(Suppl 107):53-55, 1995.
39. Hirsch JI, Tisnado J, Cho S-R et al. Use of isosulfan blue for identification of lymphatic vessels: experimental and clinical evaluation. AJR 139:1061-1064, 1982.

Table 1. Summary of Results of SLND in Breast Cancer Using Three Methods

SLND Method	N	Sentinel Node Identification Rate (%)	Accuracy (%)	False Negative Rate (%)
Blue Dye Only				
Giuliano[13]	174	66	96	12
Guenther[18]	145	71	97	10
Giuliano[14]	107	94	100	0
Koller[19]	98	98	97	3
Flett[20]	68	82	95	14
Dale[21]	21	66	100	0
Radioguided Only				
Krag[25]	443	§91	97	11
De Cicco[30]	250	96	97.5	2.5
Veronesi[23]	163	98	98	5
Borgstein[26]	130	94	99	2
Crossin[27]	50	84	98	2.4
Miner[28]	42	98	98	2.4
Offodile[29]	41	98	100	0
Pijpers[24]	37	92	100	0
Krag[22]	22	82	100	0
Combined Technique				
Cox[17]	466	94	*NR	*NR
Albertini[31]	62	92	100	0
O'Hea[33]	59	93	95	15
Barnwell[34]	42	90	100	0
Borgstein[32]	33	100	100	0

§93% had a hot spot identified; in 8 of these, the sentinel node was not found.
*NR= not recorded as not all patients received ALND if sentinel node was negative for metastases.

3

POSTMASTECTOMY RADIOTHERAPY

Abram Recht, MD
Associate Professor of Medicine
Department of Radiation Oncology, Harvard Medical School
Beth Israel Deaconess Medical Center

INTRODUCTION

Postmastectomy radiotherapy (PMRT) clearly reduces the risk of local-regional failure (LRF) for patients with invasive breast cancer. However, for many years it has been controversial whether or not this reduction also results in decreased risks of distant failure and, ultimately, death due to cancer. This was largely because randomized trials employing PMRT without systemic therapy did not show improved survival, compared to surgery alone,[1-6] with the exception of one trial.[7] However, simultaneous publication in the *New England Journal of Medicine* in October 1997 of two trials routinely employing chemotherapy suddenly brought this debate renewed life.[8,9] These studies showed that giving radiation therapy following modified radical mastectomy not only reduced LRF rates but also yielded clinically-relevant improvements in disease-free and overall survival rates.

This chapter will review the randomized trials in which PMRT has been used in conjunction with systemic therapy. Some published studies have also shown lower risks of LRF than in the global populations of the Danish and British Columbia trials. Therefore, I will discuss whether the results in randomized trials are representative of others' experiences. Finally, I will discuss how to put these findings into perspective, compared to the results achieved with other oncologic technologies. Further discussion of the issues raised here may be found elsewhere.[10-12]

RESULTS OF POSTMASTECTOMY
RADIOTHERAPY IN RANDOMIZED TRIALS

A large number of randomized trials have compared systemic therapy to systemic therapy plus radiotherapy in (predominantly) node-positive patients treated with modified radical mastectomy. All trials reporting LRF rates showed that PMRT substantially reduced the risk of such failure (by roughly two-thirds to three-quarters, proportionally). With regards to relapse-free and overall survival rates, the chance that a benefit was shown appeared related to the trial size. In studies with fewer than 200 evaluable patients, sometimes the control arm fared better,[13-15] sometimes the PMRT arm did.[16-18] In addition, discrepancies were seen within studies, in that sometimes the relapse-free survival rate would be improved in the PMRT arm but the overall survival rate was superior in the systemic-therapy only arm, or vice-versa.[15,17,19] Seven of the 8 trials containing 200 or more patients showed trends favoring the PMRT arm, with absolute improvements of 2-17% in recurrence-free and 2-11% in overall survival rates in the irradiated cohort.[8,9,20-24] (The exception was the ECOG Stage III trial.)[25] Of note, the trend for improved results with PMRT was found whether chemotherapy or tamoxifen was used as the systemic therapy (Table 1).

The proportional and absolute improvements in relapse-free and overall survival were substantial in the two largest trials which have been fully published to date. In the Danish trial of premenopausal patients, PMRT reduced the odds of any recurrence or death by 41% and the relative risk of death from any cause by 29% on multivariate analysis. The 10-year relapse-free and overall survival rates in the PMRT arm were 48% and 54%, respectively, compared to 34% and 45% in the control arm, respectively.[8] In the British Columbia trial, the reduction in the relative risk of any recurrence at 15 years was 33% and the reduction in the risk of death due to any cause by 26%. The 15-year relapse-free and overall survival rates in the PMRT arm were 50% and 54%, respectively, compared to 33% and 46% in the control arm, respectively.[9]

The Early Breast Cancer Trialists' Collaborative Group conducted a meta-analysis which did not show an advantage in overall survival at 10 years for patients receiving PMRT following surgery, compared to those who did not.[4] However, the analysis included trials in which breast-conserving surgery, simple mastectomy, or radical mastectomy, as well as modified radical mastectomy, were used. In addition, many of the included trials employed outdated radiotherapy techniques, such as the use of orthovoltage equipment. Most importantly, the trials were not segregated in which systemic therapy was routinely given to patients from those in which systemic therapy was used. A meta-analysis using published data from 11 trials (involving 4942 patients) in which all patients received systemic therapy showed that, in 8 of 11 trials, the use of PMRT reduced mortality, with an overall mortality odds ratio of 0.80 (95% confidence interval, 0.71-0.89, $p = 0.0001$).[26]

Much of the debate regarding the value of PMRT has centered around patients thought to be at "low" risk of LRF, particularly those with 1-3 positive axillary nodes. It is important to note that PMRT improved outcome in both the Danish and British Columbia studies in patients with 1-3 involved nodes as effectively (in proportional terms) as for patients with 4 or more involved nodes. For example, the 10-year disease-free and overall survival rates among the 545 patients with 1-3 positive nodes in the PMRT arm of the Danish trial were 54% and 62%, respectively, compared to 39% and 54%, respectively, among the 516 patients in the control arm. The 10-year disease-free and overall survival rates among the 248 patients on the PMRT with 4 or more positive nodes were 27% and 32%, respectively, compared to 14% and 20% among the 262 patients in the control arms, respectively.[8] In the British Columbia trial, overall survival rates in these subgroups were not reported. However, the rates of systemic failure at 15 years among patients with 1-3 positive nodes were 37% and 51% in the PMRT (91 patients) and control arms (92 patients), respectively; in patients with 4 or more positive nodes, the rates were 67% and 80%, respectively (with 58 and 54 patients in these groups, respectively).[9]

Improvements in disease-free and overall survival rates favoring the irradiated patients were also found in the Danish trial within subgroups defined by patient age (except for survival among the patients age 50-59), tumor size, the number of removed axillary nodes, the frequency of positive nodes, the histopathologic classification of the tumor (except for survival medullary carcinomas), and histologic grade.

FACTORS INFLUENCING LOCAL-REGIONAL
FAILURE RATES FOLLOWING MASTECTOMY

There is marked variability in the reported rates of LRF in patients treated with mastectomy and systemic therapy. These range from approximately 15-40%.[11] One reason for the variability may be the use of different systems for scoring events, varying lengths of follow-up, differing tumor-related characteristics of the study populations, and substantial variability in treatment techniques (both systemic and surgical). For example, some investigators do not score patients who present with such sites of disease with simultaneous evidence of distant relapse. (For example, few series report the incidence of local-regional failure developing following the development of distant metastases.)[23] When the broader definition of LRF is used, including patients with simultaneous distant failure, the rate of LRF will be about one-third higher than when using the more restrictive definition. Only 80% of LRF following mastectomy are seen within 5 years of surgery in most series with longer follow-up.[27] In the British Columbia trial a substantial proportion of the observed local-regional failures occurred more than 10 years after treatment.[9] Hence the length of follow-up will substantially affect the observed results.

Patient populations also differ between the reported series in ways which may impact the observed rates of LRF. The most important such factor may be the extent of axillary nodal involvement. In general, the risk of LRF is lower for patients with 1-3 positive nodes than for patients with 4 or more positive nodes. However, even when adjusting for this factor, LRF rates still vary substantially. For example, LRF rates in patients with 1-3 involved nodes in the Danish trial[8] (crude rate of 30%) and British Columbia trial[9] (10-year actuarial rate of 16% but 15-year actuarial rate of 33%) were substantially higher than in the few other published series with more than 5 years of follow-up which have reported results according to the number of involved nodes (6-13%).[28-30] Similar discrepancies may be noted for patients with 4 or more positive nodes between results in these two trials (crude rate of 42%, and 10- and 15-year actuarial rates of and 41% and 46%, respectively) and those of other investigators (14-24%).[22, 28-31]

Other tumor-related factors besides axillary nodal status which might affect the risk of local-regional failure include: tumor size; the presence of vascular or lymphatic invasion;[32] tumor grade;[32-34] HER-2 oncogene expression;[35] p53 expression;[36] and the distance of tumor from the pectoralis fascia.[37-39]

Only a few published studies have examined the risk of LRF in clinically-relevant subgroups defined by *combinations* of axillary nodal status and other prognostic factors. These have focussed on the results in subgroups defined by tumor size (T1 versus T2 versus T3,[33] or T1-2 versus T3)[40,41] combined with the number of involved nodes (negative nodes, 1-3 positive nodes, and 4 or more nodes[41] or 4-7 positive nodes and 8 or more positive nodes).[40,41] Such combinations were more prognostic than single factors alone. However, none of these studies gave results according to actual tumor size (e.g., < 1 cm, 1-2 cm, 2-3 cm, etc.), nor was nodal status further subdivided (e.g., 1 positive node, 2 nodes, etc.). Further, all three studies scored only isolated LRF. Follow-up time was also short — only recurrences within the first three years of follow-up were reported. Two series also included some patients who did not receive any systemic therapy.[33,40] A recent study examined the correlates of LRF for patients with 10 or more positive axillary nodes.[42] The number of involved nodes and tumor size both exerted statistically significant effects on this risk in a multivariate analysis, while patient age and estrogen-receptor protein level did not. However, the actual rates of failure in such patient subgroups were not described.

An analysis has recently been performed of 2016 unirradiated patients entered onto 4 randomized trials conducted by the Eastern Cooperative Oncology Group (ECOG).[43] The median follow-up time for patients without recurrence was 12.1 years. The first site of failure was: isolated LRF, 254 (13%); LRF with simultaneous distant failure, 166 (8%); and distant only, 679 (34%). The total risk of LRF at 10 years was 13% in patients with 1 to 3 positive nodes and 29% for patients with 4 or more positive nodes. Multivariate analysis showed that tumor size, the number of involved nodes, estrogen receptor protein status, and the number of nodes examined were significant for the endpoint of total LRF. Patient age and menopausal status were not significant factors for either endpoint.

The extent of axillary dissection has influenced the risk of LRF in other series also. For example, in the unirradiated patients in the Danish trial 82b comparing chemotherapy to chemoradiotherapy, 133 patients who had an axillary dissection from which only 0-3 nodes were recovered had a LRF rate of 40%, compared to 32% among the 511 patients in whom 4-9 nodes were recovered and 27% for the 211 patients in whom 10 or more nodes were removed.[8] The location of the recurrences in these subgroups was not reported, however.

Chemotherapy regimens that are commonly employed today vary little from one another in their effectiveness in preventing LRF. For example, CMF-based and doxorubicin-based regimens appeared about equally effective in this regard in the NSABP B-15 and SWOG 8313 trials.[44,45] Adding doxorubicin to CMF did not decrease the risk of LRF in a study conducted in Milan (although data were not separately presented for patients treated with mastectomy or breast-conserving therapy).[46] Whether more recent innovations in chemotherapy, such as adding taxanes or using very high-dose programs, will reduce LRF rates compared to "standard" regimens remains to be determined. However, increasing the dose-intensity of cyclophosphamide did not decrease LRF rates in the NSABP B-22 trial.[47]

The duration of tamoxifen use may also be important with regards to its impact on LRF. Although very short programs of tamoxifen (one year or less) appear to have some effect on LRF rates,[48] longer courses may be better. For example, a trial performed in postmenopausal node-positive patients (ECOG Trial 4181) showed a decreased incidence of LRF in patients receiving 5 additional years of tamoxifen following 12 cycles of CMFPT (4%), compared to patients receiving either only 4 cycles (8%) or 12 cycles (11%) of chemohormonal therapy at a median follow-up time of 4.1 years.[49] However, the optimal duration of tamoxifen therapy with regards to this endpoint is uncertain. Several studies have shown no substantial difference in LRF rates between patients who received at least 2 years of tamoxifen and those receiving longer courses.[50-52]

There are few data from randomized trials directly comparing LRF rates in patients treated with hormone therapy, compared to chemotherapy or combined chemohormonotherapy. In the Italian GROCTA Trial I, which enrolled both pre- and postmenopausal patients with node-positive, ERP-positive tumors, the incidences of isolated local-regional failure (including patients treated with breast-conserving therapy) in patients receiving tamoxifen for 5 years, chemotherapy, or both were 12%, 13%, and 5%, respectively, at a median follow-up time of 5 years.[53] Similar reductions in LRF rates for node-positive patients age 50 or older with estrogen-receptor or progesterone-receptor positive tumors were seen in the NSABP B-16 trial, although with shorter follow-up.[54] However, no difference in LRF rates were seen in similar patients assigned to 2 years of tamoxifen (20%) or tamoxifen plus 8 cycles of intravenous CMF (18%) in the MA.4 trial conducted by the National Cancer Institute of Canada.[55] Nor did adding oophorectomy to CMFP reduce LRF rates for premenopausal patients entered on the IBCSG Trial II.[56]

DISCUSSION

Patients with cancer often consider benefits of even less than 5% in long-term survival rates sufficiently attractive to undergo chemotherapy, whereas unafflicted health-care professionals and members of the community do not.[57,58] The same appears true for irradiation after breast-conserving surgery. In a survey conducted in Hamilton, Ontario, 78 of 82 patients (95%) with early-stage invasive cancers chose to be irradiated rather than observed.[59] In a study in Toronto, breast cancer patients were generally willing to forgo irradiation only when the absolute reduction in the risk of recurrence was less than 1%.[60] Patients who had undergone radiotherapy at the Joint Center for Radiation Therapy following conservative surgery also felt such treatment was worthwhile, even if it had limited benefits.[61] It seems likely that patients faced with a decision to undergo PMRT will seek similar minimum levels of benefit. Given that the potential long-term complications of PMRT and radiotherapy for patients treated with breast-conserving therapy are similar,[62] patients are likely to find the benefits of treatment outweigh the risks, even for situations with relatively low expected rates of LRF.

Many commonly-used oncologic therapies also result in small absolute improvements in long-term survival rates, comparable to those seen in the PMRT trials — for example, a 4-5% increase in the 5-year survival rate in patients with non-small cell lung cancer treated with chemotherapy,[63] a 6.6% increase in the 10-year survival rate for node-negative patients with estrogen-receptor positive or unknown breast cancers receiving tamoxifen for 5 years,[64] or a 7.1% improvement in the 10-year survival rate for node-negative breast cancer patients younger than 50 years treated with chemotherapy.[65]

All subgroups analyzed in both the Danish and British Columbia trial benefitted from irradiation with regards to improved disease-free and overall survival rates. Nonetheless, certain node-positive subgroups of patients may well have such low LRF rates in some institutions that patients will not routinely find the benefits sufficient or clearly-enough proven to undergo such treatment, when weighed against the potential side-effects of radiotherapy. However, I believe that at present such decisions should be based on the premise that irradiation is more likely than not to be of benefit.

CONCLUSIONS

Postmastectomy radiotherapy clearly reduces the risk of LRF for patients with invasive breast cancer with involved axillary lymph nodes. For many years it has been controversial whether or not it also decreases the risks of distant failure and, ultimately, death due to cancer, especially for patients receiving systemic therapy. There is now clear evidence that PMRT confers such benefits. However, published series vary substantially in describing the incidence of LRF following mastectomy with regards to particular patient subsets (such as those defined by the number of involved axillary nodes). Details of surgery and systemic therapy also affect this risk. Much remains uncertain with regards to the benefits of postmastectomy radiotherapy in specific situations. Nonetheless, it appears that perhaps the majority of node-positive patients will benefit sufficiently from PMRT to make its use a commonplace once again.

REFERENCES

1. Cuzick J, Stewart H, Rutqvist L, et al: Cause-specific mortality in long-term survivors of breast cancer who participated in trials of radiotherapy. J Clin Oncol 12:447-453, 1994.
2. Recht A: The return (?) of postmastectomy radiotherapy (Editorial). J Clin Oncol 13:2861-2864, 1995.
3. Harris JR, Morrow M: Local management of invasive breast cancer, in Harris JR, Lippman ME, Morrow M, et al (eds): Diseases of the Breast. Philadelphia, J.B. Lippincott, 1996, pp 485-545.
4. Early Breast Cancer Trialists' Collaborative Group: Effects of radiotherapy and surgery in early breast cancer: an overview of the randomized trials. N Engl J Med 333:1444-1455, 1995.
5. Pierce LJ, Lichter AS: Defining the role of post-mastectomy radiotherapy: the new evidence. Oncology (Huntingt) 10:991-1002, 1996.
6. Fowble B: Postmastectomy radiotherapy: then and now. Oncology (Huntingt) 11:213-239, 1997.
7. Arriagada R, Rutqvist LE, Mattsson A, et al: Adequate locoregional treatment for early breast cancer may prevent secondary dissemination. J Clin Oncol 13:2869-2878, 1995.
8. Overgaard M, Hansen PS, Overgaard J, et al: Postoperative radiotherapy in high-risk premenopausal women with breast cancer who receive adjuvant chemotherapy. N Engl J Med 337:949-955, 1997.
9. Ragaz J, Jackson SM, Le N, et al: Adjuvant radiotherapy and chemotherapy in node-positive premenopausal women with breast cancer. N Engl J Med 337:956-962, 1997.
10. Recht A, Bartelink H, Fourquet A, et al: Postmastectomy radiotherapy: questions for the twenty-first century. J Clin Oncol 16:2886-2889, 1998.
11. Recht A: Local-regional failure rates in patients with involved axillary nodes following mastectomy and systemic therapy. Semin Radiat Oncol 9:223-229, 1999.
12. Recht A: Postmastectomy loco-regional radiotherapy: is it here to stay? Semin Oncol 2000 (in press).
13. Blomqvist C, Tiusanen K, Elomaa I, et al: The combination of radiotherapy, adjuvant chemotherapy (cyclophosphamide-doxorubicin-ftorafur) and tamoxifen in Stage II breast cancer. Long-term follow-up results of a randomized trial. Br J Cancer 66:1171-1176, 1992.
14. Hayat H, Brufman G, Borovik R, et al: Adjuvant chemotherapy and radiation therapy vs. chemotherapy alone for Stage II breast cancer patients (Abstr.). Ann Oncol 1 (suppl.):21, 1990.

15. Griem KL, Henderson IC, Gelman R, et al: The 5-year results of a randomized trial of adjuvant radiation therapy after chemotherapy in breast cancer patients treated with mastectomy. J Clin Oncol 5:1546-1555, 1987.

16. Schulz K-D, Reusch K, Schmidt-Rhode P, et al: Consecutive radiation and chemotherapy in the adjuvant treatment of operable breast cancer, in Salmon SE, Jones SE (eds): Adjuvant Therapy of Cancer III. New York, Grune & Stratton, 1982, pp 411-418.

17. Muss HB, Cooper MR, Brockschmidt JK, et al: A randomized study of chemotherapy (L-PAM vs CMF) and irradiation for node positive breast cancer: eleven year follow-up of a Piedmont Oncology Association trial. Breast Cancer Res Treat 19:77-84, 1991.

18. Klefström P, Gröhn P, Heinonen E, et al: Adjuvant postoperative radiotherapy, chemotherapy, and immunotherapy in Stage III breast cancer. Cancer 60:936-942, 1987.

19. Gervásio H, Alves H, Rito A, et al: Phase III study: adjuvant chemotherapy versus adjuvant radiotherapy plus chemotherapy in women with node-positive breast cancer (Abstr.). Breast J 4 (suppl. 1):S88, 1998.

20. Ahmann DL, O'Fallon JR, Scanlon PW, et al: A preliminary assessment of factors associated with recurrent disease in a surgical adjuvant clinical trial for patients with breast cancer with special emphasis on the aggressiveness of therapy. Am J Clin Oncol 5:371-381, 1982.

21. McArdle CS, Crawford D, Dykes EH, et al: Adjuvant radiotherapy and chemotherapy in breast cancer. Br J Surg 73:264-266, 1986.

22. Vélez-García E, Carpenter JT, Moore M, et al: Postsurgical adjuvant chemotherapy with or without radiotherapy in women with breast cancer and positive axillary nodes: a South-Eastern Cancer Study Group (SEG) trial. Eur J Cancer 28A:1833-1837, 1992.

23. Tennvall-Nittby L, Tenegrup I, Landberg T: The total incidence of loco-regional recurrence in a randomized trial of breast cancer TNM Stage II: the South Sweden Breast Cancer Trial. Acta Oncol 32:641-646, 1993.

24. Overgaard M, Hansen PS, Overgaard J, et al: Randomized trial evaluating postoperative radiotherapy in high-risk postmenopausal breast cancer patients given adjuvant tamoxifen. Results from the DBCG 82c trial (Abstr.). Radiother Oncol 48 (suppl. 1):S78, 1998.

25. Olson JE, Neuberg D, Pandya KJ, et al: The role of radiotherapy in the managment of operable locally advanced breast cancer: results of a randomized trial by the Eastern Cooperative Oncology Group. Cancer 79:1138-1149, 1997.

26. Whelan T, Wright J, Julian J, et al: Does radiation therapy post-mastectomy improve survival? A meta-analysis (Abstr.). Breast Cancer Res

Treat 50:286, 1998.

27. Recht A, Hayes DF, Eberlein TJ, et al: Local-regional recurrence after mastectomy or breast-conserving therapy, in Harris JR, Lippman M, Morrow M, et al (eds): Diseases of the Breast. Philadelphia, J.B. Lippincott, 1996, pp 649-667.

28. Goldhirsch A, Gelber RD, Castiglione M: Relapse of breast cancer after adjuvant treatment in premenopausal and perimenopausal women: patterns and prognoses. J Clin Oncol 6:89-97, 1988.

29. Buzdar A, McNeese MD, Hortobagyi GN, et al: Is chemotherapy effective in reducing the local failure rate in patients with operable breast cancer? Cancer 65:394-399, 1990.

30. Kaufmann M, Jonat W, Abel U, et al: Adjuvant randomized trials of doxorubicin/cyclophosphamide versus doxorubicin/cyclophosphamide/ tamoxifen and CMF chemotherapy versus tamoxifen in women with node-positive breast cancer. J Clin Oncol 11:454-460, 1993.

31. Chu AM, Kiel K: Comparison of adjuvant postoperative radiotherapy and multiple-drug chemotherapy (CMF-VP) in operable breast cancer patients with more than four positive axillary lymph nodes. Cancer 50:212-218, 1982.

32. O'Rourke S, Galea MH, Morgan D, et al: Local recurrence after simple mastectomy. Br J Surg 81:386-389, 1994.

33. Pisansky TM, Ingle JN, Schaid DJ, et al: Patterns of tumor relapse following mastectomy and adjuvant systemic therapy in patients with axillary lymph node-positive breast cancer. Cancer 72:1247-1260, 1993.

34. Bijker N, Rutgers EJT, Peters JL, et al: Modified radical mastectomy or how to achieve optimal loco-regional control in larger breast cancers (Abstr.). Eur J Surg Oncol 20:258, 1994.

35. Stal O, Sullivan S, Wingren S, et al: c-erbB-2 expression and benefit from adjuvant chemotherapy and radiotherapy of breast cancer. Eur J Cancer 31A:2185-2190, 1995.

36. Zellars RC, Clark GM, Allred DC, et al: Prognostic value of p53 for local failure in mastectomy treated breast cancer patients (Abstr.). Proc Am Soc Clin Oncol 17:104a, 1998.

37. Ahlborn TN, Gump FE, Bodian C, et al: Tumor to fascia margin as a factor in local recurrence after modified radical mastectomy. Surg Gynecol Obstet 166:523-526, 1988.

38. Mentzer SJ, Osteen RT, Wilson RE: Local recurrence and the deep resection margin in carcinoma of the breast. Surg Gynecol Obstet 163:513-517, 1986.

39. Freedman GM, Fowble BL, Hanlon AL, et al: A close or positive margin

after mastectomy is not an indication for chest wall irradiation except in women aged fifty or younger. Int J Radiat Oncol Biol Phys 41:599-605, 1998.

40. Fowble B, Gray R, Gilchrist K, et al: Identification of a subgroup of patients with breast cancer and histologically positive axillary nodes receiving adjuvant chemotherapy who may benefit from postoperative radiotherapy. J Clin Oncol 6:1107-1117, 1988.

41. Sykes HF, Sim DA, Wong CJ, et al: Local-regional recurrence in breast cancer after mastectomy and adriamycin-based adjuvant chemotherapy: evaluation of the role of postoperative radiotherapy. Int J Radiat Oncol Biol Phys 16:641-647, 1989.

42. Diab SG, Hilsenbeck SG, deMoor CA, et al: Radiation therapy and survival in breast cancer patients with 10 or more positive axillary lymph nodes treated with mastectomy. J Clin Oncol 16:1655-1660, 1998.

43. Recht A, Gray R, Davidson NE, et al: Local-regional failure ten years following mastectomy in patients with histologically involved axillary lymph nodes receiving adjuvant chemotherapy with or without tamoxifen without irradiation: experience of the Eastern Cooperative Oncology Group. Submitted for publication.

44. Fisher B, Brown AM, Dimitrov NV, et al: Two months of doxorubicin-cyclophosphamide with and without interval reinduction therapy compared with 6 months of cyclophosphamide, methotrexate, and fluorouracil in positive-node breast cancer patients with tamoxifen-nonresponsive tumors: results from the National Surgical Adjuvant Breast and Bowel Project B-15. J Clin Oncol 8:1483-1496, 1990.

45. Budd GT, Green S, O'Bryan RM, et al: Short-course FAC-M versus 1 year of CMFVP in node-positive, hormone receptor-negative breast cancer: an Intergroup study. J Clin Oncol 13:831-839, 1995.

46. Moliterni A, Bonadonna G, Valagussa P, et al: Cyclophosphamide, methotrexate, and fluorouracil with and without doxorubicin in the adjuvant treatment of resectable breast cancer with one to three positive axillary nodes. J Clin Oncol 9:1124-1130, 1991.

47. Fisher B, Anderson S, Wickerham DL, et al: Increased intensification and total dose of cyclophosphamide in a doxorubicin-cyclophosphamide regimen for the treatment of primary breast cancer: findings from the National Surgical Adjuvant Breast and Bowel Project B-22. J Clin Oncol 15:1858-1869, 1997.

48. Castiglione M, Gelber RD, Goldhirsch A: Adjuvant systemic therapy for breast cancer in the elderly: competing causes of mortality. J Clin Oncol 8:519-526, 1990.

49. Falkson HC, Gray R, Wolberg WH, et al: Adjuvant trial of 12 cycles of CMFPT followed by observation or continuous tamoxifen versus four cycles of CMFPT in postmenopausal women with breast cancer: an Eastern Cooperative Oncology Group phase III study. J Clin Oncol 8:599-607, 1990.

50. Tormey DC, Gray R, Falkson HC: Postchemotherapy adjuvant tamoxifen beyond five years in patients with lymph node-positive breast cancer. J Natl Cancer Inst 88:1828-1833, 1996.

51. Current Trials Working Party of the Cancer Research Campaign Breast Cancer Trials Group: Preliminary results from the Cancer Research Campaign trial evaluating tamoxifen duration in women aged fifty years or older with breast cancer. J Natl Cancer Inst 88:1834-1839, 1996.

52. Swedish Breast Cancer Cooperative Group: Randomized trial of two years versus five years of adjuvant tamoxifen for postmenopausal early stage breast cancer. J Natl Cancer Inst 88:1543-1549, 1996.

53. Boccardo F, Rubagotti A, Amoroso D, et al: Chemotherapy versus tamoxifen versus chemotherapy plus tamoxifen in node-positive, oestrogen-receptor positive breast cancer patients. An update at 7 years of the 1st GROCTA (Breast Cancer Adjuvant Chemo-hormone Therapy Cooperative Group) Trial. Eur J Cancer 28:673-680, 1992.

54. Fisher B, Redmond C, Legault-Poisson S, et al: Postoperative chemotherapy and tamoxifen compared with tamoxifen alone in the treatment of positive-node breast cancer patients aged 50 years and older with tumors responsive to tamoxifen: results from the National Surgical Adjuvant Breast and Bowel Project B-16. J Clin Oncol 8:1005-1018, 1990.

55. Pritchard KI, Paterson AHG, Fine S, et al: Randomized trial of cyclophosphamide, methotrexate, and fluorouracil chemotherapy added to tamoxifen as adjuvant therapy in postmenopausal women with node-positive estrogen and/or progesterone receptor-positive breast cancer: a report of the National Cancer Institute of Canada Clinical Trials Group. J Clin Oncol 15:2302-2311, 1997.

56. International Breast Cancer Study Group: Late effects of adjuvant oophorectomy and chemotherapy upon premenopausal breast cancer patient. Ann Oncol 1:30-35, 1990.

57. Slevin ML, Stubbs L, Plant HJ, et al: Attitudes to chemotherapy: comparing views of patients with cancer with those of doctors, nurses, and general public. Br Med J 300:1458-1460, 1990.

58. McQuellon R, Muss H, Hoffman S, et al: The influence of toxicity on treatment preferences of women with breast cancer (Abstr.). Proc Am Soc Clin Oncol 13:76, 1994.

59. Whelan TJ, Levine MN, Gafni A, et al: Breast irradiation postlumpectomy: development and evaluation of a decision instrument. J Clin Oncol 13:847-853, 1995.

60. Palda VA, Llewellyn-Thomas HA, Mackenzie RG, et al: Breast cancer patients' attitudes about rationing postlumpectomy radiation therapy: applicability of trade-off methods to policy-making. J Clin Oncol 15:3192-3200, 1997.

61. Hayman JA, Fairclough DL, Harris JR, et al: Patient preferences concerning the trade-off between the risks and benefits of routine radiation therapy after conservative surgery for early-stage breast cancer. J Clin Oncol 15:1252-1260, 1997.

62. Shapiro CL, Recht A: Late effects of adjuvant therapy for breast cancer. J Natl Cancer Inst Monogr 16:101-112, 1994.

63. Non-small Cell Lung Cancer Collaborative Group: Chemotherapy in non-small cell lung cancer: a meta-analysis of updated data on individual patients from 52 randomized clinical trials. BMJ 311:899-909, 1995.

64. Early Breast Cancer Trialists' Collaborative Group: Tamoxifen for early breast cancer: an overview of the randomized trials. Lancet 351:1451-1467, 1998.

65. Early Breast Cancer Trialists' Collaborative Group: Polychemotherapy for early breast cancer: an overview of the randomized trials. Lancet 352:930-942, 1998.

66. Martinez A, Ahmann D, O'Fallon J, et al: An interim analysis of the randomized surgical adjuvant trial for patients with unfavorable breast cancer (Abstr.). Int J Radiat Oncol Biol Phys 10 (suppl. 2):106, 1984.

67. Schmoor C, Bastert G, Bojar H, et al: Effect of radiotherapy in addition to 6 cycles CMF in node positive breast cancer patients (Abstr.). Eur J Cancer 34 (suppl. 5):S59, 1998.

Table 1. Randomized Trials Comparing Systemic Therapy to Systemic Therapy Plus Radiotherapy Following Modified Radical Mastectomy

Trial/Years/Refs	FU	Results
Danish BCG 82c, 1982-89[24]	?	Crude (?) rates for LRF (± simultaneous DM) as first site of failure, 10-yr actuarial rates for RFS and OS: Group # Pts LRF RFS OS T 689 35%* 24%* 36%* T+RT 686 8% 35% 45%
South Sweden, 1978-85[23]	96	Crude rates (for LRF, at any time during follow-up incl. following DM): Group # Pts LRF RFS T 244 18%* 61% T+RT 239 6% 69%
Danish BCG 82b, 1982-89[8]	114	Crude rates as first site of failure for LRF (± simultaneous DM); 10-yr actuarial rates for RFS and OS: Group # Pts LRF* RFS* OS* CT 856 32% 34% 45% CT+RT 652 9% 48% 54% CT: 0 N+ 77 17% 62% 70% CT-RT: 0 58 3% 74% 82% CT: 1-3 N 516 30% 39% 54% CT+RT: 1-3 545 7% 54% 62% CT: 4+LN 262 42% 14% 20% CT+RT: 4+ 248 14% 27% 32%
British Columbia, 1978-86[9]	150	15-yr actuarial rates (LRF without simultaneous DM): Group # Pts LRF RFS OS CT 154 33%* 33%* 46% CT+RT 164 13% 50% 54% CT: 1-3 N 92 33% CT+RT: 1-3 91 10% CT: 4+LN 54 46% CT+RT: 4+ 58 21% Rates of LRF and systemic disease reported for nodal subgroups, but not total RFS or OS. Rates of systemic failure (CT vs. CT+RT): 1-3 LN – 51% vs. 37%; 4+ LN – 80% vs. 67%.

SEG, 1976-81[22]	120	Crude rates (as first site of failure for LRF only; excl. simultaneous LRF+DM): Group # Pts LRF RFS OS CT 176 23%* 38%* 44% CT+RT 117 13% 51% 55%
South Sweden, 1978-85[23]	96	Crude rates (at any time during follow-up for LRF, incl. following DM): Group # Pts LRF 6% 63% CT 139 17%* RFS 65% CT+RT 148 OS not reported.
Glasgow, 1976-82[21]	63	Crude LRF (as first site of failure, excl. simultaneous LRF+DM) and OS; actuarial 5-yr RFS: Group # Pts LRF RFS OS CT 108 25%* 43%* 57% CT+RT 111 11% 51% 61%
Mayo Clinic, 1974-?[20,66]	>48	Crude results for LRF as first site of failure (not stated whether incl. simultaneous LRF+DM); 5-yr actuarial RFS and OS (from 1984 abstract): Group # Pts LRF RFS OS CT 104 30%* 48% 66% CT+RT 108 10% 53% 68%
DFCI 74122, 1974-84[15]	53	Crude failure rates (LRF±DM), as assigned: Group # Pts LRF Relapse Deaths CT 100 17%* 38% 28% CT+RT 106 7% 39% 34% Crude failure rates (LRF excludes pts with DM more than 1 mo after dx of LRF), as assigned: Group # Pts LRF Relapse Deaths MF/CMF 40 2% 25% 15% MF/CMF + RT 43 5% 21% 23% AC 60 20%* 47% 37% AC + RT 63 6% 51% 41%

German BSG, 1984-89[67]	96	Relative risks (RT, 98 pts vs no-RT, 101 pts) with 95% confidence intervals reported; no absolute results reported for each arm separately. LRF (not defined): RR 0.35 (0.14-0.91)* RFS: RR 0.82 (0.55-1.21) Distant failure: RR 1.01 (0.65-1.57) OS: RR 0.93 (0.62-1.40)

Piedmont 74176, 1976-?[17]		Crude LRF (±DM); actuarial 10-yr RFS and OS:

Group	# Pts	LRF	RFS	OS
L-PAM	43	35%	41%	48%
L-PAM-RT	33	18%	58%	61%
CMF	44	16%	50%	58%
CMF-RT	39	8%	45%	46%
No RT	87	25%	45%	53%
RT	72	13%	51%	53%

Crude recurrence by # involved nodes and regimen:

Group	L-PAM	L+RT	CMF	C+RT
1-3 N+	39%	47%	25%	50%
	(9/23)	(7/17)	(6/24)	(10/20)
4+ N+	85%	50%	75%	58%
	(17/20)	8/16)	(15/20)	(11/19)

Israel, 1981-83[14]	?	Rate (not stated if crude or actuarial) of LRF (±DM): CT (58 pts): 24%; CT+RT (54 pts): 4% "No statistical difference" in 5-yr RFS, but data not provided Survival (from [4]): CT: 71%; CT+RT: 61%

Helsinki-Tampere, 1981-84[13]	90	Actuarial 5-yr LRF (±DM); actuarial 8-yr RFS and OS:

Group	# Pts	LRF	RFS	OS
CT	52	24%	56%	69%
CT + RT	47	7%	56%	65%

MD Anderson 7730B[4]	?	Crude OS: CT (54 pts): 55%; CT + RT (43 pts): 35%

Köln, Germany, 1976-?[16]	36	Actuarial 3-yr RFS (estimated from figure) and crude OS (no data on LRF):

Actuarial 3-yr RFS (estimated from figure) and crude OS (no data on LRF):

Group	# Pts	RFS	OS
AC	28	68%	16%
AC + RT	43	84%	4%

Helsinki, 1976-81[18]	?	Crude 5-year LRF (±DM) and RFS; actuarial 5-yr OS (estimated from figure); levamisole and no-levamisole arms combined

Crude 5-year LRF (±DM) and RFS; actuarial 5-yr OS (estimated from figure); levamisole and no-levamisole arms combined

Group	# Pts	LRF	RFS	OS
CT	40	58%	18%	68%
CT + RT	39	13%*	59%*	90%*

ECOG, 1982-87[25]	109	Crude results (LRF±DM):

Crude results (LRF±DM):

Group	# Pts	LRF	Relapse	Deaths
CT	148	24%*	56%	53%
CT + RT Received	164	15%	60%	54%
RT Refused	134	10%	58%	?
RT	30	40%	70%	?

LRF (±DM) in pts: receiving RT-10% (13/134); refusing RT, but randomized

*: P-value <0.05 between the irradiated and unirradiated arms.
Abbreviations:
CT: chemotherapy arm
CT + RT: chemotherapy plus radiotherapy arm
FU: median follow-up time, in months
L and L-PAM: l-phenylalanine mustard
LRF: local-regional recurrence
OS: overall survival
RFS: relapse-free survival
T: tamoxifen
?: not stated

4

The Molecular and Cellular Biology of HER2/*neu* Gene Amplification/ Overexpression and the Clinical Development of Herceptin (Trastuzumab) Therapy for Breast Cancer

Mark D. Pegram, M.D.
Adjunct Assistant Professor of Medicine
Division of Hematology Oncology
UCLA School of Medicine

Gottfried Konecny, M.D.
Post-Graduate Research Fellow
Division of Hematology Oncology
UCLA School of Medicine

Dennis J. Slamon, M.D.
Professor and Chief
Division of Hematology Oncology
UCLA School of Medicine

INTRODUCTION

Proto oncogenes represent a family of genes which when activated have been shown to play a role in the pathogenesis of a number of malignancies in vertebrate species including humans.[1,2] In physiologic states these same genes are known to play a role in the normal cell growth control and differentiation. The HER2/*neu* gene is a member of the Type I receptor tyrosine kinase (RTK) group which is one of the subfamilies in the proto oncogene family and encodes a 185kD surface membrane receptor protein. This gene has been localized to chromosome 17q21,[1] and the encoded protein is expressed in a wide variety of tissues including the skin, oral mucera, breast, ovary, endometrium, lung, liver, pancreas, small and large bowel, kidney, bladder and the central nervous system as well as some connective tissues.[4-5] The exact physiological role of the HER2/*neu* protein in these tissues is not completely understood, but like other proto oncogenes it is believed to play an important signaling role in cellular proliferation and differentiation processes. Current data suggests that it forms hetero-dimers with other members of the RTKI family (such as HER 1, HER3 and HER4 in response to various ligands known as heregulins.[6-8] Activation of HER2/*neu* results in an increase its kinase activity which in turn initiates signal transduction resulting in either cellular proliferation and/or differentiation, depending on the ligand as well as the conditions.[9-14] In human breast cancers, a non-inherited alteration occurs in this gene in 25-30% of cases. This alteration is gene amplification resulting in as many as 50 to 100 gene copies per cell rather than the normal two copies of the gene per cell (one on each chromosome 17).[15-17] This amplification event results in overexpression of p185$^{HER2/neu}$ at both the transcript and protein levels, such that there can be as many as ~2,000,000 HER2/*neu* molecules per cell in malignant tissues, instead of the normal ~20,000 - 50,000 molecules per cell. Again this alteration is the result of a somatic (non-inherited) event occurring sometime during the life of the patient for reasons that are still unclear. When the HER2/*neu* gene is overexpressed at these abnormally high levels, however, its kinase activity is similarly increased, possibly due to autoactivation caused by crowding of adjacent HER2/*neu* receptor molecules within the cell membrane.[9] The net result appears to be ligand-independent activation of p185$^{HER2/neu}$ resulting in an increase in mitogenic cell signaling increased cell proliferation. There is now substantial published data demonstrating that this molecular alteration is associated with a poor clinical prognosis in early stage breast cancer in terms of a shortened disease free interval, as well as shortened overall survival.[15,16] Initially this finding was controversial with many published studies failing to demonstrate an association between HER2 gene amplification and clinical outcome; but in retrospect, it is clear that most of these contradictory studies were due to a number of methodologic problems, including the fact that the reagents and/or methods used to detect HER2 overexpression were insensitive or that the studies were statistically underpowered (small sample sizes) or had too short a duration of clinical follow-up.[18] It is now clear, using good reagents and methodologies, in large cohorts with sufficient clinical follow-up (some as much as 30 years), that HER2 overexpression is an independent prognostic factor predicting poor clinical outcome, increasing the relative risk of relapse by a factor of 2-7 fold depending on amount of amplification/overexpression for both node positive as well as node negative breast cancers.[19,20]

A significant body of basic science and clinical data demonstrate that HER2/*neu* overexpression, plays an important role in the pathophysiology of these malignancies containing the alteration. Cells with HER2/*neu* overexpression have an increase in cell proliferation, an increase in anchorage-independent cell growth, an increase in tumorigenicity, and an increase in metastatic potential as compared to control cells lacking HER2/*neu* overexpression (Figure 1). Since HER2/*neu* overexpression and its accompanying increase kinase activity is at least in part driving the tumors aggressive biological behavior, it is a logical target for therapeutic intervention by antibodies or other molecules which can suppress or otherwise alter the effects of the HER2 kinase on cell signaling.

Figure 1. MCF7 breast carcinoma cells engineered to overexpress HER2 proliferate at nearly twice the rate of control (NEO) MCF7 cells

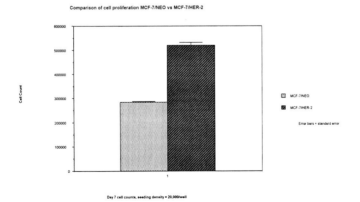

Identification of the HER-2 Alteration in
Human Breast Cancer Specimens

As stated above, one of the early problems in the HER-2/*neu* field as it relates to breast cancer resulted from the variable and sometimes inappropriate or inaccurate methods used to detect the alteration. Despite a number of current marketing claims, detection of the HER-2/*neu* alteration is still not completely accurate using a number of the commercially available tests including and especially the FDA approved Herceptest from DAKO. Many of these assays are suboptimal for detection of the HER-2/*neu* alteration. The approaches have been used to detect HER2 gene amplification at the DNA level have included slot blot or Southern blot, fluorescence *in situ* hybridization or PCR-based techniques. Overexpression has been measured at the transcript level using Northern analysis or RT-PCR, or at the protein level using Western blot, immunohistochemistry, or ELISA assays. It is clear that all of the solid matrix blotting techniques suffer from potential dilutional artifacts resulting from the admixture of normal stromal, inflammatory and vascular cells which do not contain the alteration, with malignant cells in clinical tumor samples.[16,22] Techniques involving *in situ* detection are thought to be more sensitive in identifying gene amplification or protein overexpression since by definition they circumvent this problem. The most widely used technique for detection of HER2 overexpression at the protein level is immunohistochemistry. The problem with this technique is that a wide variety of primary antibodies are currently in clinical use, each of which has differing sensitivity and specificity, as well as variable cutoff values to distinguish overexpressing form non-overexpressing tumors.[18] As a result it is therefore difficult to know whether a sample scored as HER2 positive in one laboratory will be confirmed as HER2 positive by another laboratory. Another concern is that the degree of immunohistochemical staining for HER2 is subjective and qualitative. It is clear that formalin fixation of tumor samples and storage in paraffin can result in epitope degradation so that sensitivity is lost over time in archival clinical material.[16] To lessen this problem, some assays resort to a technique called antigen retrieval which consists of heating the tumor sample using a number of methods including microwave radiation, water baths, ovens, etc. in order to "retrieve" epitopes that have been lost during tissue fixation, embedding and storage. This approach, however, can create new problems in that normal tissues and non-HER2-overexpressing malignancies which contain normal physiologic levels of HER2 expression also have enhancement of the signal from a normal amounts of HER2 protein and results in a false positive interpretation of HER2 overexpression. Recent reports from a number of groups suggest a higher than expected false positive rate using the FDA-approved HercepTest[TM] for detection of HER2 overexpression, and this is most likely due to the antigen retrieval step used in this assay.[23,24] The ELISA assay to detect soluble HER2 protein in serum samples is not practical as a diagnostic assay for early stage breast cancer, since soluble HER2 protein seems to be found in the serum of patients with either high disease burden and/or high level HER2 overexpression, such as in cases of metastatic disease.[25] For patients with small primary tumors, this assay is almost always negative even if the tumor overexpresses HER2 at the tissue level.

The most accurate technique currently available for detection of HER2 gene alteration appears to be DNA-fluorescence *in situ* hybridization (FISH).[20,22] This assay uses a fluorescent labeled genomic DNA probe containing the HER2 gene and its flanking sequence which is hybridized to the DNA within the tumor cells in standard paraffin embedded tumor section mounted on a microscope slide. A second DNA probe, specific for chromosome 17 centromere and labeled with a different color, is used to distinguish true HER2 gene amplification versus increased HER-2/*neu* signals resulting from chromosome 17 ploidy. Using this technique, the number of HER2 genes per chromosome 17 centromere can be quantitated. One theoretical disadvantage of this assay is the inability to detect the so called "single copy overexpressors." In such cases, the HER2 protein is overexpressed in the absence of HER2 gene amplification.[22] However, the frequency of single copy HER2 overexpression in breast cancers is estimated to be less than 5% of all overexpressing tumors. Moreover, these cases do not appear to have the poor prognosis of the amplified/overexpressors, therefore the advantages of FISH in terms of sensitivity and specificity far outweigh this single disadvantage in terms of diagnostic accuracy.[22,26] The other potential problem with FISH methodology is its current general availability and cost. These problems will lessen with the recent approval of FISH technology for HER2 analysis by the FDA. It is likely that cost will decrease with the increased economy of scale of HER2 testing using this technique and it is already becoming more broadly available.

It is critical to remember that HER2 overexpression correlates well with a number of other established prognostic factors and clinical parameters in breast cancer (Table 1). Therefore a clinician may be able to estimate the probability that a particular breast tumor will harbor HER2 overexpression based on these clinical parameters. If the results of a particular HER2 diagnostic assay are inconsistent with the clinical picture (particularly if an immunoassay was used for the HER2 analysis) then a different assay methodology should be used to retest the sample to confirm or refute the initial result. For example, a high grade, lymph node positive, ER-negative tumor, with a high S-phase fraction and aneuploidy, is consistent with a HER2 positive phenotype, especially if the patient relapses quickly. By contrast, a node-negative, diploid, ER-positive, well differentiated breast carcinoma with low S-phase is not likely to be HER2 positive. Another important clinical observation is that HER2 overexpression is rarely seen in lobular carcinomas. Thus despite the availability of sophisticated molecular diagnostic tools, solid clinical judgment as always, still applies.

Table 1. Association of HER2 Overexpression with Other Clinicopathologic Variables

• high S-phase fraction
• aneuploidy
• absence of ER/PR expression
• presence of nodal metastasis
• high nuclear grade
• short relapse-free interval
• ductal (as opposed to lobular) histology

Development of Herceptin

Soon after HER2 receptor alteration was shown to play a role in the pathogenesis of aggressive human breast cancer, efforts were made to identify and characterize inhibitors of HER2 which might interrupt its pathogenic activity. To date numerous agents have been identified which target HER2 such as: tyrosine kinase inhibitors, inhibitors of various constituents of the ras signaling pathway, heregulin-toxin fusion proteins, single chain antibodies, HER2 antisense molecules, small molecule receptor antagonists, and monoclonal antibodies. Of these, one particular murine monoclonal antibody, 4D5, was found to have significant and dose dependent efficacy specifically against HER2-overexpressing cancer cells, while having no effect on cells expressing physiologic levels of HER2.[27]   Prior murine monoclonal antibodies against numerous tumor targets tested in a number of clinical trials in the past, proved negative.   There were a number of reasons for this including the development of human anti-murine antibodies (HAMA), which rapidly neutralize murine antibodies rendering them useless as far as anti-tumor activity is concerned. New breakthroughs in biotechnology (specifically gene sequence engineering) have allowed the possibility of overcoming this limiting clinical problem.   Murine monoclonal antibodies can now be "humanized" by identifying the minimum set of amino acid residues in the complementarity determining region (CDR) of the murine antibody required for antigen specificity and antigen binding affinity, and substituting these regions into the CDRs of a consensus human IgG framework.[21]   Maintaining both antigen specificity and binding affinity through this process is a painstaking exercise, however it is essential to finding a humanized variant with desired specifications.   Ultimately, antibody humanization was achieved for the murine 4D5 anti HER-2/*neu* monoclonal antibody (by Genentech, Inc.), resulting in a recombinant, humanized monoclonal antibody directed against HER2 (rhuMAb HER2). This drug is now known as Herceptin.[28]   The specificity of 4D5 for the HER2 protein was maintained during this engineering process, and the binding affinity (kD ~0.1nM) of the humanized variant was actually slightly improved over that of 4D5 parent molecule (Kd ~0.3nM).[28]   In addition, the Fc portion of Herceptin is based on an IgG1 consensus sequence allowing for the possibility of antibody-mediated cellular cytotoxicity against tumor target cells by immune effector cells expressing Fc receptors.[29]   More importantly, preclinical studies conducted in our laboratory as well as at Genentech, demonstrated that the antiproliferative effects of 4D5, and the dose-dependent anti-tumor efficacy against HER2-overexpressing xenografts in athymic mice were also maintained following antibody humanization.[30]

Based on this demonstration of preclinical efficacy both the murine monoclonal and subsequently the humanized version were initially taken into humans in a series of single dose and multi-dose phase I clinical trials at UCLA. These trials were designed to study tumor localization, toxicology, and pharmacokinetics of single dose and multidose antibody administered IV to patients with HER2-positive, refractory, metastatic breast cancer. The murine antibody had a favorable pharmacokinetic and pharmacodynamic profile as well as very favorable toxicity (essentially none).   The only problem is that as predicted, patients formed human anti-mouse antibodies against the murine antibody.   The humanized version was tested next and the conclusions from these studies are summarized in Table 2. The Phase I studies showed that

Herceptin has a favorable pharmacokinetic profile – achieving trough serum concentrations above the concentration needed for maximal antiproliferative effects *in vitro*; and Herceptin has a limited toxicology profile with the most frequent problem being fevers during the first infusion and pain at sites of metastasis. For the most part, these symptoms were described as mild or moderate. Furthermore, there was no evidence of human anti-humanized antibodies against Herceptin. This was in contrast to a phase I trial conducted with murine 4D5 antibody in which HAMA developed rapidly, (within 12 weeks) in most treated patients.

Table 2. Conclusions from phase I Clinical Trials of Herceptin

• defined pharmacokinetics with a long serum half life achieving desired serum trough concentrations
• favorable toxicology profile (low grade fevers)
• no evidence of human anti-mouse antibodies (HAMA)
• demonstration of tumor localization with radio-iodinated 4D5

Combining Herceptin with Cytotoxic Chemotherapy: Receptor-Enhanced Chemosensitivity

Used alone, Herceptin is not cytotoxic either *in vitro* or *in vivo* for most HER-2 overexpressing breast cancer cells at least over short term exposure. HER2 positive human breast cancer cells undergo cell cycle arrest with accumulation in the G0/G1 phase of the cell cycle after treatment with Herceptin, but there is no evidence of apoptosis or cytotoxicity during short term (days) exposure and only occasionally after prolonged exposure.[29,31] One popular method of rendering antibodies cytotoxic envisioned by researchers in the anti-cancer antibody field is to covalently link cytotoxic drugs to therapeutic monoclonal antibodies. In one such effort, anti-EGF receptor (HER1) antibodies were coupled to cisplatin and tested against HER1 expressing xenografts *in vivo*.[32] As controls for this experiment, the investigators also tested uncoupled, free anti-EGFR antibodies given concomitantly with free cisplatin. What resulted was surprising in that this combination had more anti-tumor activity than the covalently linked species and much more than either drug used alone. Because of the close homology between EGFR and HER2, we conducted similar experiments in our laboratory and found the identical result with the anti-HER2 antibody plus cisplatin.[31] Furthermore, we studied the nature of the interaction between anti-HER2 and cisplatin using a well established method to test for drug interactions, and we found the combination to be highly synergistic.[31] The mechanism of synergy in this case was a HER2 antibody-mediated attenuation of DNA repair activity resulting in the accumulation of platinum-DNA adducts in the nucleus and a significant enhancement of cytotoxicity due to cisplatin, specifically in the HER-2/*neu* overexpressing cells.[31] We have termed this effect Receptor Enhanced Chemosensitivity (REC) as it applies to both the HER1 and HER2 systems. We have now expanded our antibody/drug interaction studies to include combinations of Herceptin with antimetabolites, alkylating agents, taxanes, topoisomerase II inhibitors, vinca alkaloids, and anthracyclines. Of these we have found the platinum analogs, ionizing radiation, docetaxel, vinorelbine, etoposide, and thiotepa in decreasing order to have synergistic cytotoxicity with Herceptin (Table 3).[33] One drug, 5-fluorouracil is antagonistic with Herceptin. The mechanism of this antagonistic interaction remains unknown but is the subject of ongoing investigation.

Table 3.

Drug	Interaction with Herceptin
Cisplatin/Carboplatin	Synergistic
Ionizing Radiation	Synergistic
Docetaxel	Synergistic
Vinorelbine	Synergistic
Etoposide	Synergistic
Thiotepa	Synergistic
Doxorubicin	Additive
Vinblastine	Additive
Paclitaxel	Additive
Methotrexate	Additive
5-Fluorouracil	Antagonistic

Phase II Herceptin Clinical Trials

To date, four phase II clinical trials of single agent Herceptin or Herceptin in combination with cisplatin have been conducted. In a pilot phase II study of single agent Herceptin for patients with HER2-overexpressing breast cancer who failed prior chemotherapy for metastatic disease, an 11% response rate was observed.[34] In an expanded phase II study of Herceptin as a single agent for patients who had failed one or two prior chemotherapeutic regimens for metastatic disease a 14% response rate was subsequently reported.[35] Results from single agent Herceptin given as first line therapy for HER2 positive metastatic breast cancer were more recently reported.[36] In this study a higher response rate of ~25% was observed suggesting that single agent Herceptin may be more effective in patients less heavily pretreated with chemotherapy. In addition, this study randomized patients to two different dose levels of Herceptin. The first dose level was the standard 4mg/kg loading dose followed by 2mg/kg/week, while the second was double the standard dose (8mg/kg load + 4mg/kg/week). No apparent difference in response rate was seen at the higher dose level, and the higher dose appeared to cause more frequent side effects.[36] A significant contribution from all of these studies is a better understanding of the toxicology of Herceptin. For the most part Herceptin is very well tolerated when administered as a single agent. Approximately 30-40% of patients experience fevers and/or chills during the initial (4mg/kg) loading dose of Herceptin.[28] These reactions, though sometimes dramatic due to the rigors, can easily be managed by administration of Tylenol, Benadryl, or Demerol, and/or by slowing the rate of Herceptin infusion. Other commonly reported side effects of single agent Herceptin are shown in Table 4.

Table 4.

Common side effects of single agent Herceptin (first infusion)	
fever/chills	asthenia
nausea/vomiting	diarrhea
pain at site of tumor	headache

Similar to the preclinical research, the first trial of the combination of Herceptin with chemotherapy in a clinical setting was performed at UCLA in 1992.[37] A unique feature of this phase II trial was that to gain entry into the study, all patients were required to have chemoresistant breast cancer as defined by objective evidence of disease progression (25% or greater increase in measurable disease) during active chemotherapy treatment. The study population consisted of heavily pretreated, advanced breast cancer patients with HER2 overexpression. Patients in the study were treated with a loading dose of 250mg IV Herceptin, followed by weekly doses of 100mg IV for 9 weeks. Chemotherapy consisted of cisplatin ($75mg/m^2$) on days 1, 29 and 57. Clinical response data in this study were confirmed by an independent, blinded, response evaluation committee. Objective partial clinical responses were seen in 24% of patients, and an additional 24% had either minor response (<50% shrinkage of measurable disease) or disease stabilization. This compares extremely favorably to either single agent cisplatin which has a reported response rate in five separate clinical trials of approximately 7% or less, 95% confidence limits, 2 - 11%, or single agent Herceptin which is ~12% in pretreated patients with metastatic disease.[34,37] In this study, the concomitant administration of cisplatin chemotherapy had no effect on Herceptin pharmacokinetics. The cisplatin/Herceptin study was also the first comprehensive analysis of the relationship between Herceptin pharmacokinetics and serum levels of a soluble form of the HER2 protein. The extracellular domain of p185[HER2] is cleaved from the surface of tumor cells and then measured by a serum based ELISA assay. There is a clear inverse relationship between serum soluble HER2 protein and Herceptin through concentration.[37] It has been suggested that soluble HER2 protein may be a marker of clinical response to Herceptin, however, our initial results from an admittedly small data set, demonstrate that a decrease in HER2 serum levels is not always associated with an objective clinical response. An increase in soluble HER2 protein, however, was associated with disease progression in a majority of patients in the phase II program, suggesting that this may be a useful clinical marker to estimate probability of disease progression.[37] Pretreatment serum HER2 levels did not correlate with objective clinical response to Herceptin. Finally, a very important conclusion of this study was that Herceptin did not appear to increase toxicity of cisplatin chemotherapy over that expected for cisplatin alone in this patient population. This is important since renal epithelial cells are known to express HER2 protein at normal levels and therefore were at risk for cisplatin induced renal damage.

First Line Chemotherapy Plus Herceptin for
HER2-Overexpressing Metastatic Breast Cancer

A large, prospective randomized controlled trial of standard chemotherapy, either alone or in combination with Herceptin has been completed.[38]   This trial was conducted in 469 patients with HER2-overexpressing metastatic breast cancer who had not previously been treated with chemotherapy for metastatic disease. Standard chemotherapy consisted of doxorubicin 60mg/m^2 (or epirubicin 75mg/m^2) plus cyclophosphamide 600mg/m^2 IV every 21 days for anthracycline naive patients (N = 281), or paclitaxel 175mg/m^2 IV over 3 hours for those patients who had previously been treated with an anthracycline in the adjuvant setting (N = 188). A feature of the patient characteristics for this cohort was that the patients in the paclitaxel arm had worse prognostic features at diagnosis as might be anticipated given their prior adjuvant treatment with an anthracycline. Patients on the paclitaxel arm were more likely to be premenopausal, have ER/PR, negative tumors more positive lymph nodes, a higher incidence of prior radiation treatment, and ~20% had been treated with myeloablative chemotherapy followed by peripheral blood or bone marrow-derived hematopoietic stem cell support. These patients also had a shorter time from diagnosis to relapse compared to patients treated on the doxorubicin/cyclophosphamide arm.   Based on these pretreatment characteristics, one might expect that the response to treatment in the paclitaxel group would be lower than the response to doxorubicin/cyclophosphamide-treated group in this study.   However, even with this caveat, the response rate in the paclitaxel group was somewhat of a surprise to many in that single agent paclitaxel resulted in only a 15% objective response compared to 38% for the doxorubicin-containing arm.   Patients randomized to receive Herceptin in combination with conventional chemotherapy had a higher overall response rate, a longer median response duration, a significantly longer time to disease progression, and an increase in survival at two years.[38,39]   These data which have been presented publicly, demonstrate that with a median follow-up of 29 months, Herceptin combined with either chemotherapy regimen decreased the relative risk of death by 24% and increased median survival from 20.3 months to 25.4 months.[39] This is particularly noteworthy given the fact that two thirds of the women on the chemotherapy alone arms subsequently received Herceptin, at the time of disease progression, on a companion study protocol following initial protocol treatment. It is also noteworthy that Herceptin, the first biologic agent to be approved by the FDA for breast cancer treatment, prolongs survival of metastatic breast cancer patients.

Along with the clinical success of Herceptin came an unexpected toxicity: cardiac dysfunction especially for those patients who received concomitant Herceptin and doxorubicin. The incidence of Herceptin-associated cardiotoxocity was also significantly increased in the paclitaxel/Herceptin-treated group.[38] The mechanism(s) of this unique toxicity currently remains unknown. Expression of HER2 in adult myocardium was not previously well characterized, although it was presumed to be very low or absent on the basis of low level HER2 transcript expression by PCR analysis, and undetectable levels of protein expression by immunohistochemistry. Two patients at UCLA who developed clinically symptomatic congestive heart failure had endomyocardial biopsy performed as part of their diagnostic evaluation. Both of these patients had pathological findings consistent with doxorubicin-associated myocardial cell damage by both ordinary light microscopy or electron microscopy (unpublished observation). Most of the patients with this syndrome had improvement in symptoms and /or an increase in left ventricular ejection fraction (LVEF) following treatment with ACE inhibitors, diuretics, or cardiac glycosides. Clearly, all patients receiving Herceptin should undergo baseline assessment of cardiac function and periodic monitoring of LV function, and if a significant decrease in LVEF is noted, the drug should be discontinued unless there is an eminent risk of death from progressive cancer, which, in exceptional cases, may outweigh the risks of heart failure. The drug, therefore, should be used cautiously or even avoided altogether in cases of known underlying serious cardiac illness, at least until the mechanism of cardiotoxicity is better defined, and/or until pretreatment risk factors for cardiotoxicity can be studied and understood more completely.

Future Clinical Development of Herceptin

At the time of this writing there are a number of unknown questions regarding the potential clinical applications of Herceptin in cancer therapy. For example, the precise mechanism of action of Herceptin is still incompletely understood. Although inroads into this question are being made, to date there is still no direct experimental evidence from clinical studies that confirm that Herceptin is a true immunotherapeutic. The optimum duration of Herceptin therapy is also currently unknown. The clinical trials performed to date have been conducted with Herceptin treatment until the time of disease progression. Would shorter duration of Herceptin be as efficacious? Or conversely, would continued Herceptin treatment beyond the time of progression in fact slow the rate of progression? Whether or not Herceptin will have activity in other malignancies is not yet known, but a number of trials are either already underway or about to begin in multiple malignancies including ovarian cancer, non-small cell lung cancer, prostate cancer, colon cancer, gastric cancer and many others. The preclinical studies would predict that Herceptin efficacy is likely to be restricted to cancers that exhibit amplified/overexpression of HER-2/*neu*. The initial clinical data seem to support this, however, the question is yet to be completely resolved. The integration of Herceptin with standard chemotherapy, hormonal therapy, and radiation therapy remains an active area of research. Clinical trials of a number of chemotherapy drug combinations with Herceptin are planned or underway.

The use of adjuvant Herceptin for HER-2 positive early stage breast cancer is a very attractive treatment approach from both a theoretical and practical point of view. As Herceptin is a therapeutic with a high molecular weight (~150kD), penetration of the antibody into bulky tumor deposits is unfavored due to the high interstitial oncotic pressure and poor vascularization within metastatic solid tumors as well as the CNS due to the blood/brain barrier. Therefore, efficacy of Herceptin should theoretically be maximal in a micrometastatic disease situation where intratumoral pharmacokinetic boundaries do not apply as much and at which time CNS involvement may not have occurred. Large scale studies of adjuvant Herceptin for breast cancer are now beginning. These studies will require careful designing to avoid the cardiotoxicity issues surrounding the use of Herceptin/anthracycline administration. This is a difficult problem given the fact that anthracyclines have now become a mainstay of adjuvant therapy and there is evidence that HER2-positive patients may benefit from anthracycline based therapy.[40-42] Most of the adjuvant studies will use one year of adjuvant Herceptin, but the decision for this duration of Herceptin administration, though reasonable, is entirely empiric. With the recognition of the cardiotoxicity potential we have proposed a non-anthracycline adjuvant chemotherapy/Herceptin regimen consisting of docetaxel/platinum combination which will avoid anthracycline-associated cardiotoxicity issues in the adjuvant setting where many women may be cured as a result of their initial surgery and radiation. More importantly, however, this approach will take advantage of the observed and documented synergy between these agents. Whether or not Herceptin has activity in non-HER2 overexpressing breast cancers is an important issue which is being addressed in a number of ongoing clinical trials. Once again the scientific rationale for this approach is completely absent. The optimal dosing schedule and route of administration of Herceptin continues to be studied. Because Herceptin has a long serum half life, it lends itself to less frequent administration such as using twice the standard dose every other week. Formulations of Herceptin are also being pursued which may allow for subcutaneous administration of the drug. Data from our laboratory indicate that efficacy of Herceptin is maintained when given subcutaneously in mouse models (unpublished observation). Very little is known about Herceptin resistance, but clearly such mechanisms must exist since many breast cancer patients treated with the drug do not in fact have an objective clinical response. A better understanding of such mechanisms might allow for improved treatment approaches to HER2 positive breast cancers.

Many clinical issues regarding HER2 amplification/overexpression remain unresolved. Its use as a prognostic factor, its use as a predictive marker for response to conventional breast cancer therapies, and its use as a target for future drug development provide a wealth of opportunities for future basic and clinical research. The fact that Herceptin prolongs survival of patients with metastatic breast cancer is not only clinically significant for breast cancer therapy, but it also is the ultimate experimental proof from a scientific perspective that HER2 does play an important role in the pathophysiology of breast cancer, a fact which has long been disputed by investigators, a number of whom are now vocal proponents but who sharply criticized clinical application of the early laboratory investigations on HER2 biology, and who dismissed and/or rejected the concept of HER2-targeted cancer therapeutics with monoclonal antibodies. The HER2 paradigm of targeted cancer therapy is now an important model for drug discovery and drug development in the biotechnology and pharmaceutical industries. Based on the experience with Herceptin we believe that there will be other molecules that, like HER2, will be the targets for future novel cancer treatments. These new cancer therapeutic targets will require validation through careful scientific studies conducted in the laboratory, and through carefully designed clinical trials. It is certain, however, that identification of new therapeutic targets will result in significant therapeutic benefits for future patients suffering from breast cancer as well as most other human malignancies. The coming decade should prove quite exciting with substantive advances in diagnosis, treatment and ultimately prevention being a definite payoff of the basic science knowledge base which the field of cancer research has and will continue to produce.

REFERENCES:

1. Slamon, D.J. Proto-oncogenes and human cancers. N Engl J Med 317:955-957, 1987.
2. Slamon, D.J. Oncogenes and human malignancy, pp 226-229. In: Cline, M.J. Moderator. Oncogenes: Implications for the diagnosis and treatment of cancer. Ann Int Med 101:223-233, 1984.
3. Shih C, Padhy L, Murray M, *et al.*, Transforming genes of carcinomas and neuroblastomas introduced into muonse fibroblasts. Nature 1981; 260: 261-264.
4. Coussens L, Yang-Feng TL, Liao YC, *et al.*, Tyrosine kinase receptor with extensive homology fo EGF receptor shares chromosomal location with neu oncogene. Science 1985; 230: 1132-1139.
5. King CR, Kraus MH, Aaronson SA. Amplification of a novel v-erb-B-2-related gene in human mammary carcinoma. Science 1985; 229:974-6.
6. Carraway K, Cantley L. A neu acquaintance for erbB3 and erbB4: a role for receptor heterodimerization in growth signaling. Cell 1994;78:5-8.
7. Sliwkowski M, Schaefer G, Akita R, et al., Coexpression of erB2 and erbB3 proteins reconstitutes a high affinity receptor for heregulin. J Biol Chem 1994;269:15661-14665.
8. Plowman G, Culouscou J-M, Whitney G, et al., Ligand-specific activiation of HER4/p180erB4, a fourth member of the epidermal growth factor receptor family. Proc Natl Acad Sci USA 1993;90:1746-1750.
9. Reese DM and Slamon DJ. HER-2/neu Signal Transduction in Human Breast and Ovarian Cancer. Stem Cells 1997;15:1-8.
10. Wen D, Suggs SV, Karunagaran D, et al. Structural and functional aspects of the multiplicity of neu differentiation factors. Molecular and Cellualr Biology 14: 1909-1919, 1994.
11. Wen D, Peles E, Cupples R, et al. Neu differentiation factor: a transmembrane glycoprotein containing and EGF domain and an immunoglobulin homology unit. Cell 69: 559-572, 1992.
12. Falls, DL, Rosen KM, Corfas G, et al. ARIA, a protein that stimulates acetylcholine receptor synthesis, is a member of the neu ligand family. Cell 72: 801, 1993.
13. Marchionni M, Goodearl A, Chen M, et al. Glial growth factors are alternatively spliced erbB2 ligands expressed in the nervous system. Nature 362: 312, 1993.

14. Peles E, Ben-Levy R, Tzahor E, et al. Cell-type specific interaction of neu differentiation factor (NDF/heregulin) with neu/HER-2 suggests complex ligand-receptor relationships. EMBO J. 12: 961-971, 1993.

15. Slamon DJ, Clark GM, Wong SG, et al., Human breast cancer: correlation of relapse and survival with amplification of the HER-2/neu oncogene. Science 1987;235:177-182.

16. Slamon DJ, Godolphin W, Jones LA, et al., Studies of HER-2/neu proto-oncogene in human breast and ovarian cancer. Science 1989;244:707-712.

17. Seshadri R, Firgaira FA, Horsfall DJ, McCaul K, Setlur V, Kitchen P: Clinical significance of HER-2/neu oncogene amplification in primary breast cancer. The South Australian Breast Cancer Study Group. J Clin Oncol 11:1936-1942, 1993.

18. Press MF, Hung G, Godolphin W, et al., Sensitivity of HER-2/neu antibodies in archival tissue samples: potential source of error in immunohistochemical studies of oncogene expression. Cancer Res 1994;54: 2771-2777.

19. Toikkanen S, Helin H, Isola J, Joensuu H: Prognostic significance of HER-2 oncoprotein expression in breast cancer: a 30-year follow-up. J Clin Oncol 10: 1044-1048, 1992.

20. Andrulis IL, Bull SB, Blackstein ME, Sutherland D, Mak C, Sidlofsky S, Pritzker KP, Hartwick RW, Hanna W, Lickley L, Wilkinson R, Qizilbash A, Ambus U, Lipa M, Weizel H, Katz A, Baida M, Mariz S, Stoik G, Dacamara P, Strongitharm D, Geddie W, McCready D, for the Toronto Breast Cancer Study Group: neu/erbB-2 amplification identifies a poor-prognosis group of women with node-negative breast cancer. Toronto Breast Cancer Study Group. J Clin Oncol 16: 1340-1349, 1998.

21. Carter P, Presta L, Gorman CM, et al: Humanization of an anti-p185HER2 antibody for human cancer therapy. Proc Natl Acad Sci USA 89: 4285-4289, 1992.

22. Pauletti G, Godolphin W, Press MF, Slamon DJ: Detection and quantitation of HER-2/neu gene amplification in human breast cancer archival material using fluorescence in situ hybridization. Oncogene 13: 63-72, 1996.

23. Roche and Ingle, Increased HER2 with U.S. FDA-Approved Antibody J Clin Oncol 17: 434-435, 1999(letter).

24. Diane Maia, Immunohistochemical Assays for HER2 Overexpression J Clin Oncol 17: 434, 1999.

25. Pegram M, Lipton A, Hayes D, et al: Phase II Study of Receptor-Enhanced Chemosensitivity Using Recombinant Humanized Anti-p185HER-2/neu Monoclonal Antibody Plus Cisplatin in Patients With HER-2/neu-

Overexpressing Metastatic Breast Cancer Refractory to Chemotherapy Treatment. J Clin Oncol 16: 2659-2671, 1998.

26. Pegram MD, Pauletti G, and Slamon DJ., HER-2/neu as a predictive marker of response to breast cancer therapy. Breast Cancer Res and Treat 1998, 52(1-3):65-77.

27. Lewis GD, Figari I, Fendly B, Wong WL, Carter P, Gorman C, Shepard HM: Differential responses of human tumor cell lines to anti-p185[HER2] monoclonal antibodies. Cancer Immunol Immunother 37: 255-263, 1993.

28. Herceptin (Trastuzumab) anti-HER2 monoclonal antibody: product package insert, Genentech, Inc. South San Francisco, CA, copyright September, 1998.

29. Pegram MD, Baly D, Wirth C, et al., Antibody dependent cell-mediated cytotoxicity in breast cancer patients in Phase III clinical trials of a humanized anti-HER2 antibody. Proc Am Assoc Cancer Res 1997;38:602(abstract).

30. Pietras RJ, Pegram MD, Finn RS, et al: Remission of human breast cancer xenografts on therapy with humanized monoclonal antibody to HER-2 receptor and DNA-reactive drugs. Oncogene 17: 2235-2249, 1998.

31. Pietras RJ, Fendly BM, Chazin VR, et al: Antibody to HER-2/neu receptor blocks DNA repair after cisplatin in human breast and ovarian cancer cells. Oncogene 9: 1829-1838 , 1994.

32. Aboud-Pirak E, Hurwitz E, Pirak ME, et al: Efficacy of antibodies to epidermal growth factor receptor against KB carcinoma in vitro and in nude mice. J Natl Cancer Inst 80: 1605-1611, 1988.

33. Pegram M, Hsu S, Lewis G, et al., Inhibitory effects of combinations of HER-2/neu antibody and chemotherapeutic agents used for treatment of human breast cancers. Oncogene 18: 2241-2251, 1999.

34. Baselga J, Tripathy D, Mendelsohn J, et al: Phase II study of weekly intravenous recombinant humanized anti-p185HER2 monoclonal antibody in patients with HER2/neu-overexpressing metastatic breast cancer. J Clin Oncol 14: 737-744, 1996.

35. Cobleigh MA, Vogel CL, Tripathy D, Robert NJ, Scholl S, Fehrenbacher L, Paton V, Shak S, Lieberman G, Slamon D: Efficacy and Safety of Herceptin (Humanized Anti-HER2 Antibody) as a Single Agent in 222 Women with HER2 Overexpression who Relapsed Following Chemotherapy for Metastatic Breast Cancer. Proc Am Soc Clin Oncol 17: 376, 1998.

36. Vogel CL, Cobleigh MA, Tripathy D, et al., Efficacy and safety of Herceptin (Trastuzumab, humanized anti-HER2 antibody) as a single agent

in first-line treatment of HER2 overexpressing metastatic breast cancer (HER2+/MBC). Breast Cancer Res and Treat 1998;50:232a.

37. Pegram M, Lipton A, Hayes D, et al: Phase II Study of Receptor-Enhanced Chemosensitivity Using Recombinant Humanized Anti-p185HER-2/neu Monoclonal Antibody Plus Cisplatin in Patients With HER-2/neu-Overexpressing Metastatic Breast Cancer Refractory to Chemotherapy Treatment. J Clin Oncol 16: 2659-2671, 1998.

38. Slamon D, Leyland-Jones B, Shak S, Paton V, Bajamonde A, Fleming T, Eiermann W, Wolter J, Baselga J, Norton L: Addition of Herceptin (Humanized anti-HER-2 Antibody) to First Line Chemotherapy for HER2 Overexpressing Metastatic Breast Cancer (HER2+MBC) Markedly Increases Anticancer Activity: A Randomized, Multinational Controlled Phase III Trial. Proc Am Soc Clin Oncol 17: 377, 1998.

39. Norton L, Slamon D, Leyland-JHones B, et al., Overall Survival (OS) Advantage to Simultaneous chemotherapy (Crx) Plus the Humanized Anti-HER2 Monoclonal Antibody Herceptin (H) in HER2-Overexpressing (HER2+) Metastatic Breast Cancer (MBC). Prc Am Soc Clin Oncol 1999;18:483(abstract).

40. Muss HB, Thor AD, Berry DA, Kute T, Liu ET, Koerner F, Cirrincione CT, Budman DR, Wood WC, Barcos M, Henderson C: c-erbB-2 expression and response to adjuvant therapy in women with node-positive early breast cancer. New Engl J Medicine 330: 1260-1266, 1994.

41. Thor AD, Berry DA, Budman DR, Muss HB, Kute T, Henderson IC, Barcos M, Cirrincione C, Edgerton S, Allred C, Norton L, Liu ET: erbB-2, p53, and Efficacy of Adjuvant Therapy in Lymph Node-Positive Breast Cancer. J Natl Cancer Inst 90: 1346-1360, 1998.

42. Paik S, Bryant J, Park C, Fisher B, Tan-Chiu E, Hyams D, Fisher ER, Lippman ME, Wickerham DL, Wolmark N: erbB-2 and Response to Doxorubicin in Patients With Axillary Lymph Node-Positive, Hormone Receptor-Negative Breast Cancer. J Natl Cancer Inst 90: 1361-1370, 1998.

5

HIGH-DOSE CHEMOTHERAPY FOR BREAST CANCER

Yago Nieto, MD
Instructor

Elizabeth J Shpall, MD
Professor of Medicine
University of Colorado Bone Marrow Transplant Program

INTRODUCTION

Autologous stem cell transplantation (ASCT), using hematopoietic progenitor cells derived from either the bone marrow or peripheral blood, allows for the administration of chemotherapy (CT) with a several fold increase in the doses. The goal is to achieve a higher tumor-cell kill than standard-dose CT, in the hope that it will translate into an improvement in outcome. In the high-dose chemotherapy (HDCT) setting, extramedullary organ toxicities become dose limiting.[1] The improvement in supportive care has decreased the morbidity and mortality associated with HDCT to a current toxic death rate of less than 5%.[2]

DOSE INTENSITY AND BREAST CANCER

Following in vitro observations of dose response, retrospective analyses have shown that dose intensity of CT correlates with antitumor activity and clinical outcome, both in the metastatic[3,4] and in the adjuvant setting.[5,6] Prospective studies in metastatic breast cancer (MBC) have demonstrated that decreasing the dose below the standard range compromises the antitumor effect and palliation.[7] In contrast, trials testing minor increases in dose intensity of doxorubicin,[8] paclitaxel,[9] or epirubicin[10,11,12,13,14] in MBC have failed to show an improved outcome.

Similar results have been obtained in the adjuvant setting. A prospective randomized trial of cyclophosphamide (CPA), doxorubicin and fluorouracil (CAF) administered to node-positive patients in three dose intensity levels showed that the low level was inferior to the intermediate and high levels in aggregate, but with no significant differences in outcome between the intermediate and high dose levels.[15,16] A similar trial, comparing 50 versus 100 mg/m^2 of epirubicin within the FEC regimen (fluorouracil, epirubicin and CPA) showed improved disease-free survival (DFS) and overall survival (OS) at the higher dose arm.[17] Several adjuvant trials have compared standard doses to escalated dose of CPA,[18,19] or doxorubicin,[20] with G-CSF support. These trials have shown greater toxicity and no improvement in efficacy with this degree of dose escalation with G-CSF.

Most authors agree that these results are supportive of the concept of dose intensity within, but not above the standard-dose range. Both in the adjuvant and in the metastatic setting, there seems to be a dose threshold below which dose reductions compromise outcome, whereas modest increments increase toxicity without an added benefit.

In contrast to these strategies, HDCT with ASCT is based on the hypothesis that major dose increments are needed to overcome tumor cell resistance and produce a meaningful clinical improvement. Stem-cell support allows to increase the dose above bone marrow tolerance, in an attempt to maximally capitalize on the dose-response curve of certain antineoplastic drugs.

HDCT FOR METASTATIC BREAST CANCER (MBC)

MBC is incurable in the vast majority of patients receiving standard-dose CT.[21]

Although many patients have tumors which initially respond, CT becomes progressively less active, and eventually the disease becomes refractory to treatment.

The first HDCT trials for MBC breast cancer were initiated in the mid 1980's. As in other settings where CT is used with curative intent, these trials assumed the basic principle that minor dose reductions would critically compromise outcome,[22] and thus, that only the maximally tolerated doses (MTDs) of the drugs should be delivered. In vitro data and previous results of CT in other diseases, such as leukemia, supported the use of drug combinations over single agents.[23] Alkylating agents constituted the backbone of HDCT regimens, based on their anti-breast cancer activity, steep dose-response effect, non-cross resistance, and nonoverlapping extramedullary toxicities.[23] (Table 1)

A series of trials using HDCT as salvage treatment for refractory MBC patients produced a high response rate, never before seen with standard-dose CT in patients with resistant disease.[24,25,26,27] Responses, however, were short-lived and had no impact on survival. Results improved when HDCT was moved upfront as initial therapy for metastatic disease, with around 10-15% of patients remaining long-term free of recurrence.[28] The results initially reported by Peters et al., using the STAMP -I regimen of CPA, cisplatin and BCNU, were consistently reproduced by other groups, using similar alkylating agent-based HDCT combinations.[30,31] In a next step HDCT was used as immediate consolidation of aggressive standard-dose adriamycin-based induction CT, which was administered to maximally cytoreduce the tumor burden prior to HDCT. Phase II trials testing this strategy consistently showed that 15-25% of patients remained long-term free of disease.[29,30,31] (Table 2) Since HDCT was shown to be most effective at a time of minimal tumor burden, potent induction regimens, such as AFM (doxorubicin, fluorouracil and methotrexate),[32] were designed to provide substantial cytoredution prior to HDCT. Local treatment with surgery or radiotherapy (RT) was added posttransplant to sites of prior bulky disease. In parallel to these advances, the introduction of G-CSF posttransplant, peripheral blood progenitor cells (PBPCs) in place of bone marrow (BM), and other improvements in supportive care, reduced treatment-related mortality from the initial 15-20% rate to the current 2-4% expected in experienced transplant units.

The 15-20% fraction of chemosensitive metastatic breast cancer patients rendered long-term free of disease by HDCT in phase II studies seems substantially higher than the expected long-term DFS of 0-3%, using conventional CT.[21,33,34] These results were unheard of in prospective studies of standard-dose CT, and they generated great enthusiasm in physicians and public. The number of women receiving HDCT increased progressively and since 1992 breast cancer was the most common indication for HDCT and ASCT.[2]

Detractors of HDCT have argued that its results may be explained by patient selection (younger age, better performance status), extensive staging bias, and the requirement of proven chemosensitivity.[35,36] This controversy underscores the need for mature data from prospective, well designed and adequately sized randomized phase III trials.

On the other hand, there is a major need to improve HDCT for breast cancer. It seems unlikely that the first generation of high-dose regimens, such as STAMP-I or STAMP-V developed 15 years ago, are the optimal stem-cell supported high-dose combinations. While current randomized trials, initiated several years ago, are testing such first-generation regimens, the field needs substantial progress. Several new strategies are being actively pursued: 1) development of new HDCT combinations, 2) tandem or multiple transplants, 3) integration of HDCT into a multimodal approach, combined with novel treatments, with a different mechanism of action, against minimal residual disease.

**Which MBC Patients Are Most Likely
To Benefit from HDCT?**

While the results from phase II trials of HDCT in MBC generated great interest, it became clear that the majority of MBC patients relapsed after HDCT. Several retrospective analyses have identified favorable and unfavorable prognostic factors for outcome in this patient population. Liver metastases, prior adjuvant CT, extensive prior treatment for metastatic disease, extensive number of metastatic sites, lack of major response to pretransplant induction CT, and relapse within a prior radiation field have been identified as independent negative predictors of outcome.[37,38,39] On the other hand, a single metastatic site and pretransplant CR status, and prolonged interval from primary diagnosis to relapse seem favorable predictors.[39,40,41]

It appears that patients with poor prognostic features do not benefit from the first-generation high-dose regimens. Newer high-dose regimens or alternative high-dose strategies need to be developed in poor prognosis MBC patients seeking aggressive treatment.

Another aspect of the controversy regarding HDCT for MBC is that patients with good prognosis MBC are often not offered HDCT until their disease is extensive and refractory. The hypothesis that good prognosis MBC patients might attain major benefit from HDCT early in the course of their disease was prospectively tested at the University of Colorado.[40] A prospective phase II study of four cycles of doxorubicin-based induction followed by HDCT with STAMP-I was conducted in MBC patients with no evidence of disease (NED), defined as one or more sites of macroscopic tumor that could be either resected en bloc and/or encompassed within a single RT field, and no prior CT for metastatic disease at study entry. At a median follow-up of 49 months, DFS and OS rates were 55% and 65%, respectively, with median DFS/OS of 43/77 months (Fig.4). In the subgroup of patients with a single metastatic site, 68% remain alive with no evidence of recurrence at latest follow-up. These encouraging results in MBC patients who might be highly curable with HDCT, suggest the benefits of early detection of distant recurrences with closer follow-up after adjuvant treatment, and of early HDCT in MBC with good prognosis features.

New HDCT Regimens for MBC

A critical review of the first generation of high-dose regimens shows that there is ample room for improvement. While cisplatin and carboplatin are active drugs in first-line treatment for breast cancer,[42,43] they are only escalated twofold in STAMP-I and STAMP-V, respectively. Both regimens also include cyclophosphamide (CPA). Two recent randomized NSABP studies have shown no benefit from substantial increases in to the dose-intensity and cumulative dose of CPA, combined with doxorubicin, in the adjuvant treatment of node-positive patients. The four-fold dose-escalation of CPA achieved in these trials raises concerns about its use in high-dose regimens for breast cancer. A possible explanation for why CPA does not show an in vivo dose-response effect, in contrast to the observations in vitro using 4-hydroxy-CPA, may stem from its own pharmacology. CPA is a prodrug that requires hepatic activation to 4-hydroxy-CPA, a P450-mediated metabolic step that is subject to saturation and drug-drug interactions.[44] This activation step has a high interpatient[45] and intrapatient[46] variability. We have observed large and unpredictable intrapatient variations in CPA pharmacokinetics over the three treatment days using STAMP-I. Busse et al. studied the intrapatient changes in the metabolic pathways of CPA and its metabolites when given at standard and high doses, and observed that, at high doses, the inactivating reactions significantly increased and the bioactivation of CPA was reduced, when compared to conventional doses.[47]

Current research efforts are developing new high-dose combinations using more active drugs. While not alkylating agents, a dose-response effect has been shown with doxorubicin,[48] paclitaxel[49,50,51] and docetaxel.[52,53] The potential of doxorubicin for cardiotoxicity has precluded its inclusion in most HDCT regimens. Myelosuppression is dose limiting when paclitaxel[54] and docetaxel[55,56] are given at conventional doses. The MTD of paclitaxel, delivered in a 24-hour infusion, in combination with fixed doses of cyclophosphamide and cisplatin, with ASCT, was established at 775 mg/m^2.[57] This dose is around three-fold higher than the highest dose of paclitaxel given over 24 hours with G-CSF.[58,59,60] Paclitaxel has been subsequently incorporated into other HDCT regimens.[61,62]

Docetaxel is highly active against breast cancer, either as first-line therapy,[63,64] or against anthracycline-resistant disease,[65,66] both for soft tissue and visceral sites, including liver. A phase I trial of docetaxel in combination with melphalan and carboplatin, with ASCT, is underway at the University of Colorado.

Tandem Or Multiple Transplants for Metastatic BC

Another strategy under evaluation is based on the hypothesis that more than one cycle of HDCT is needed to eradicate the tumor. Dunphy et al.[67] used two cycles of nonmyeloablative dose-intense CPA-etoposide-cisplatin (DICEP), with 25% DFS at two years, comparable to the outcome after a single cycle of myeloablative HDCT. Rapid delivery of multiple cycles of stem-cell-supported dose-intense non-myeloablative chemotherapy has been proven to be feasible.[68,69]

The delivery of tandem cycles of myeloablative HDCT, with ASCT after both cycles, has been proven to be feasible.[70,71,72] However, the value of a second cycle of the same regimen remains unclear, since the PR to CR conversion rate decreases substantially from the first to the second cycle of HDCT.[72] Several investigators have tested the sequential use of non-cross-resistant HDCT regimens. Ayash et al.[73] treated chemosensitive breast cancer patients with melphalan followed, within a median of 35 days, by STAMP-V. At a median follow-up of 16 months after the second transplant, the 34% DFS rate appears similar to results of a single HDCT treatment. Preliminary results were reported by Bitran et al. using the reverse sequence of CPA-thiotepa followed by melphalan, with a longer median intercycle interval of 105 days.[74] The DFS rate was 56% at a median follow-up of

25 months from the first transplant. Whether the results of both studies are significantly different is unclear, given their short follow-up and the overlapping ranges of DFS rates. In addition, the phenomenon of acute in vivo resistance after HDCT has been recently described by Teicher et al.[75] These authors treated tumor-bearing mice with different sequential HDCT treatments. Tumors became resistant after the first treatment, in an inversely proportional fashion to the lengh of the interval between treatments. The longer intercycle interval in Bitran☐s study might allow the acquired drug resistance to revert.

Is Current HDCT Better Than Standard Chemotherapy for MBC?

The first results of randomized controlled trials in MBC came from a small study conducted at the University of Waterstrand, in South Africa. Bezwoda et al. randomized patients to receive 2 cycles of high-dose CPA, mitoxantrone and etoposide (HD-CNV) with ASCT, or 6-8 cycles of standard-dose CPA, mitoxantrone and vincristine (CNV), as upfront treatment for metastatic disease (Fig. 1-C).[76] Patients randomized to the high-dose arm also received intermediate-dose CPA for mobilization of stem cells. Both groups were well balanced in terms of performance status, prior adjuvant CT, and number of metastatic sites. However, there was a higher number of hormone receptor negative patients in the HDCT than in the control arm (53% and 35%, respectively). No treatment-related deaths were seen on either arm. All outcome parameters were significantly better for the high-dose than for the conventional-dose arm: RR (95% vs. 53%), CR rate (44% vs. 4%), median response duration (80 vs. 34 weeks) and median OS (90 vs. 45 weeks). A recent update of these results showed that 20% patients in the high-dose arm remained in unmaintained CR at a follow-up in excess of 5 years.[77] The short difference in duration between median duration of response and median OS has raised concerns about the follow-up and salvage treatments used, especially for the control arm. Only responding patients were given tamoxifen upon completion of CT; therefore, more patients in the high-dose arm received hormonal therapy. It has also been argued that the CR rate and duration of response in the control arm were lower than what could be expected from combination chemotherapy for previously untreated MBC, and that, in fact, prior phase II data of that same regimen were superior to the results of the phase III study.[78]. However, it is noticeable that a substantial number of studies testing doxorubicin-containing first-line CT in MBC have reported results very close to those of the control arm in this trial.[79,80,81,82,83] Although neither arm of the study used CT regimens commonly used in North America or Europe, this trial prospectively indicated higher antitumor activity and a survival advantage for the high-dose arm.

Peters et al. reported preliminary results of a randomized trial comparing immediate versus delayed HDCT in metastatic breast cancer patients in CR following standard-dose CT with doxorubicin, fluorouracil and methotrexate (AFM).[84] Of 423 enrolled patients, 98 (23%) achieved a CR and were randomized to immediate HDCT with STAMP-I, or to observation. Patients in PR were offered HDCT off study. Patients in the observation arm were offered HDCT at the time of relapse (Fig. 1.A). Median DFS was longer for patients immediately transplanted compared to those randomized to observation (11 vs. 3.6 months, p<0.01). However, patients transplanted at relapse had superior OS than those immediately transplanted (38 vs. 23 months, p<0.05). Although this trial was not designed to directly compare HDCT and standard-dose therapy, its results suggest that HDCT may improve DFS and OS in MBC patients in CR after standard-dose CT.

The results of the Philadelphia/ECOG randomized trial in chemoresponsive MBC patients were recently reported at the 1999 ASCO meeting.[85] Stadtmauer et al. initially enrolled 553 MBC patients to receive induction CT with CAF (n=507) or CMF (n=46). Of those, 303 patients (54%) achieved a PR (n=247) or a CR (n=56). Of the 303 responding patients, 199 were randomized to HDCT with STAMP-V or maintenance CMF (Fig. 1-B). Fifteen of those patients were considered ineligible after randomization, and thus, 184 were actually randomized, 139 in PR and 45 in CR. The analysis of those 184 patients (101 in the HDCT arm and 84 in the maintenance CT arm) at a median follow-up of 31 months, showed no statistically significant difference in RFS, OS or treatment-related mortality between the arms. This trial was initially designed to have an 85% power to detect a doubling in survival in the HDCT arm, assuming a 10% ineligibility rate and a 10% noncomplicance rate. The actual drop-out rates were 34% and 11% before and after randomization, respectively. The small number of patients in CR who were randomized and analyzed (n=45) confers this study only a 50% power to detect differences in RFS as large as 50% between both arms in this important subset of patients in CR. Most surprisingly, in the group of patients in PR (n=139), the CR conversion rate was higher in the maintenance CMF arm (9%) than in the STAMP-V arm (6%). The low conversion rate from PR to CR in the transplant arm of this trial is different than the vast majority of phase II trials, where PR to CR conversion rates of 20-60% are typically reported.[29,30,31]

Data from the French PEGASE-04 randomized study were also recently reported.[86] In this small trial, Lotz et al. randomized 61 MBC patients, in response after 4-6 cycles of conventional-dose anthracycline-based CT, to additional cycles of the same CT or to HDCT with CPA, mitoxantrone and melphalan. Thirteen of those patients were in CR and 48 in PR prior to randomization. Both groups were well balanced except for lung metastases (15 in the HDCT arm and 4 in the control arm) and CNS disease (2 in the HDC arm and none in the control arm). No toxic deaths were seen in either arm. Median progression-free survival time was significantly longer in the HDCT arm than in the control arm (26.9 months and 15.7 months, respectively) (p=0.04). Relapse rates were 27% (95% confidence interval, 12-42%) in the HDCT arm, and 52% (34-70%) in the HDCT and control arms, respectively. Median OS times were 36.1 months and 15.7 months in the HDCT and control arms, respectively, but this difference did not reach statistical significance (p=0.08).

HDCT FOR HIGH-RISK PRIMARY BREAST CANCER (HRPBC)

Phase II Studies in Node-Positive Patients

Many patients with high-risk primary breast cancer (HRPBC), defined by extensive axillary node involvement or inflammatory carcinoma (IBC), relapse after surgery and conventional-dose adjuvant CT.[87,88] A retrospective analysis by Hryniuk and Levine suggests that dose-intensity may have a greater impact on survival in the adjuvant setting than in patients with metastatic disease.[89]

Peters and colleagues conducted the first trial of HDCT with STAMP-I in patients with 10 or more involved axillary nodes.[90] At a median follow-up of five years, 71% of 85 evaluable patients remained free of disease.[91] Gianni et al. used a sequential single-agent approach in this patient population.[92] At a median follow-up of four years DFS was 57%, significantly better than that of those patients with 10 involved nodes who received the most effective of two standard-dose CT regimens compared in a randomized trial at the same institution,[93] using the same selection criteria and pretreatment staging as in Gianni's HDCT study.

The University of Colorado has piloted the use of HDCT in patients with 4-9 involved nodes, whose long-term DFS ranges from 45 to 76% with standard adjuvant treatment. Fifty-four patients received four cycles of standard-dose chemotherapy followed by HDCT using STAMP-I. A DFS rate of 71% was seen at a median follow-up of 31 months.[94] These results have been reproduced by other groups.[95,96] An ongoing intergroup randomized trial is comparing HDCT, as above described, to a dose-dense sequential combination of doxorubicin, paclitaxel, and cyclophosphamide with G-CSF support, designed at Memorial Sloan Kettering (Fig. 3).[97]

Inflammatory Breast Cancer

Inflammatory breast cancer (IBC) is a very aggressive form of the disease, with a five-year DFS rate of 30%, following multimodal therapy, with doxorubicin-based neoadjuvant CT, surgery and RT.[98,99] Recent phase II trials at the Dana Farber Cancer Institute[100] and the University of Colorado[101] have incorporated HDCT, in varying schedules, into the treatment of IBC. These studies included neoadjuvant doxorubicin-containing CT followed, in the Dana Farber study by STAMP-V and posttransplant mastectomy, and in the Colorado study by pretransplant mastectomy and STAMP-I. In both studies, locoregional RT, and tamoxifen for ER-positive patients were subsequently delivered. In both trials the DFS rate was >70% at 2-year follow-up (Fig.5).

Predictive Factors for Relapse after HDCT for HRPBC

We retrospectively analyzed all stage II/III patients treated at the University of Colorado with STAMP-I, who had survived transplant and had either relapsed at any time post-HDCT, or had been followed for at least two years without evidence of recurrence. This analysis included 176 patients, with a median follow-up of 45 (range, 12 to 84) months.[102] Tumor size, tumor grade, clinical IBC, ER/PR negativity, and nodal ratio (number of positive nodes divided by number of nodes sampled) were associated with relapse. No association was found between the following variables and recurrence: absolute number of positive nodes, pathogic IBC, DNA ploidy, S-phase fraction, multifocality, extensive intraductal component, vascular or lymphatic vessel invasion, involved nodes >2 cm, extranodal extension, age, menopausal status, family history, pregnancy and histologic type. In a multivariate analysis, tumor size, ER/PR combined status, and nodal ratio were independent predictors. Using these three factors and their specific weight in the multivariate analysis, the following scoring system was developed:

Score = (Nodal Ratio x 3.05) + (Tumor Size x 0.15) - (ER/PR x 1.15)
In this formula, tumor size is entered in cm, and ER/PR is assigned "1" if positive
(that is, ER and/or PR are positive) and "0" if negative (both negative). Scores 2.41
and <2.41 allocate patients to a high- or low-risk category, with risks of relapse of
65% and 11%, respectively. The differences in RFS (p<0.000001) and OS
(p<0.00005) were highly significant (Fig. 6). This model has 60% sensitivity, 90%
specificity, 65% positive predictive value, 88% negative predictive value, and 83%
accuracy. Our model was subsequently validated in an external set of 225 patients
treated at Duke University with STAMP-I and followed for a median 46 (range 4 to
127) months.

A subsequent analysis evaluated Her-2/neu overexpression and p53
mutations in the same patient population.[103] While Her-2/neu overexpression was
an independent predictor of RFS and OS, p53 mutations did not correlate with
outcome.

Somlo et al. analyzed 114 patients treated with two different HDCT
regimens at City of Hope, and found that PR negativity and IBC correlated with
risk of relapse.[104]

Is HDCT Better than Standard-Dose HRPBC?

As with MBC, uncontrolled phase II trials in this setting seemed to improve long-
term DFS, compared to historical controls treated with standard CT. It has also
been claimed that this improvement in outcome may be due to a stage-migration
phenomenon, resulting from extensive pre-HDCT staging, and to patient-selection
bias.[105,106] As mentioned above, the comparison made by Gianni et al. between their
two trials of HDCT and standard CT, using the same selection criteria and
pretreatment staging tests in both studies, strongly argues against the relevance of
these biases.

Results from small randomized phase II studies have been reported.
Rodenhuis et al. randomized 81 patients after neoadjuvant CT and surgery to one
more cycle of the same regimen or HDCT with CPA, thiotepa and carboplatin,
followed by posttransplant administration of locoregional RT and tamoxifen.[107] The
high-dose arm had a 15% (6/41) drop-out rate. An intent-to-treat analysis did not
show significant differences in DFS or OS between both arms. A major problem
with interpreting the results of this trial was the non-standard staging procedure
used to determine eligibility. Patients in this study never had a complete axillary

node dissection. Inclusion in this study was based on axillary level III involvement, determined by an infraclavicular lymph-node biopsy, and not based on the number of positive nodes. Additionally, the study was sized with an 80% power to detect a 30% difference in outcome. It is worth noting that this difference would have been greater than the overall impact of adjuvant CT for breast cancer compared to no treatment at all.

Hortobagyi et al. conducted a randomized phase II study in HRBC patients, defined by 10 nodes after upfront surgery or by 4 positive nodes after preoperative CT. Patients received 8 cycles of FAC followed by randomization to 2 cycles of DICEP versus no further CT.[108] All patients received RT and tamoxifen. At a median follow-up of 53 (range, 7 to 85) months, DFS and OS were not significantly different between both arms. This trial was prematurely closed due to slow accrual and did not have the statistical power to assess the efficacy of high versus standard dose CT. Additionally, the DICEP regimen has been proven to be nonmyeloablative [109,110] and is not considered HDCT.

Thus, neither Rodenhuis' nor Hortobagyi's studies contribute meaningfully to our understanding of whether HRPBC patients benefit or not from HDCT. They were not phase III trials designed to address this question, and were not powered to detect realistic differences between both arms.

An answer as to what merit there is to HDCT over standard-dose CT in HRPBC will come from well-designed, adequately powered phase III studies with adequate follow-up. The results of most of these studies, initiated several years ago, are either pending or are still preliminary. Peters et al. reported at the 1999 ASCO meeting a preliminary analysis of the CALGB Intergroup trial in patients with 10 positive nodes identified after standard axillary dissection.[111] Eligible patients received 4 cycles of CAF and were randomized to high-dose STAMP-I or to the same three drug combination at intermediate doses, which were approximately 30% of the doses in the high-dose arm. (Fig. 2-A) This study, designed to detect a 14% difference in RFS at 5 years, randomized a total of 783 patients. Patients relapsing on the intermediate-dose arm were eligible for subsequent HDCT. All patients were to receive locoregional RT, and, if hormone receptor-positive, tamoxifen for 5 years. At median follow-up of 37 months, only 60% of the expected number of relapses have occurred. The RFS and OS comparisons between the HDCT and control arms are inconclusive (68% vs. 64%, p=0.7; 78% vs. 80%, p=0.1). There were 29 toxic deaths in the HDCT arm, and none in the control arm. The relapse rate was higher in the intermediate-dose (32.2%) than in the high-dose group (21.6%), with non-overlapping 95% confidence intervals (27.6 to 36.9% and 17.5

to 25.6%, respectively). Since the study design called for an additional 3 years of follow-up prior to initial analysis, its current results are too immature for any meaningful conclusion.

At the same 1999 ASCO meeting, Bezwoda reported the results of a South African randomized trial in HRPBC (Fig. 2-C).[112] Eligible patients had T1-3a tumors and 10 involved nodes, or tumors >5 cm with 7 involved nodes and at least one more additional poor prognostic feature, including ER negativity or strong (two first degree relatives) family history of BC. Locoregional XRT was not required posttransplant, although both arms were balanced with respect to the number of patients who received SRT. This study randomized 154 patients to 2 cycles of high-dose CNV or 6 cycles of standard-dose CAF. At a median follow-up >5 years, there was a statistically significant improvement in relapse rate (p<0.001), RFS (<0.05) and OS (<0.05) for patients in the high-dose arm. **[Editor's Note: The Bezwoda study has come under scrutiny because of allegations of scientific misconduct.]**

A Swedish randomized trial was also presented at the 1999 ASCO meeting.[113] This study targeted HRPBC patients, defined as 8 involved nodes, or 5 involved nodes with an ER negative, high S-phase fraction tumor. The authors randomized 525 patients to 9 cycles of individually tailored FEC, or 3 cycles of conventional FEC, followed by HDCT with STAMP-V. All patients in both arms received RT and tamoxifen for 5 years. No pre-randomization staging tests were performed to exclude women with bone or bone marrow disease, and no information as to how balanced these patients were in both arms was provided at the meeting or in the abstract. Median follow-up was 23.7 months. Relapse rate, DFS and OS were not significantly different in either arm within the first two years of follow-up. There were eight toxic deaths in the control arm from secondary myelodysplastic syndrome/acute myelogenous leukemia, and two in the HDCT arm from acute toxicity.

Other large randomized trials, such as one conducted by ECOG (Fig. 2-B) in patients with 10 involved nodes or an US Intergroup trial for patients with 4 to 9 nodes (Fig. 3), have been completed or are actively accruing patients and are awaiting analysis in North America and Europe. It is important to bear in mind that the ascertainment of a potential benefit of HDCT over standard-dose CT requires mature follow-up and that premature evaluation of randomized trials can be misleading. We learned this lesson from the Parma randomized study in aggressive non-Hodgkin's lymphoma. Preliminary analyses of this study were negative,[114,115] but with the appropriate duration of follow-up its definitive analysis became positive, with 5-year DFS rates of 46% and 12% for the HDC and control arms, respectively.[116]

FUTURE DIRECTIONS OF IMPROVEMENT OF HDCT FOR BREAST CANCER

Purging of Stem-Cell Grafts

PBPCs have replaced BM as the primary source of hematopoietic progenitors for ASCT. Although tumor burden may be lower in PBPC than in BM fractions,[117] breast cancer cells can be detected in PBPC fractions of 10-40% of MBC patients, and 5-20% of stage II-III patients.[118,119,120,121,122] Detection of breast cancer cells in the BM at the time of HDCT has been correlated with an increased risk of relapse in HRPBC,[123,124] but not in MBC.[125] Most post-HDCT relapses in MBC patients occur in sites of prior disease, suggesting an insufficient cytoreductive capacity of HDCT, rather than a direct effect from tumor cells contaminating the graft. Thus, the clinical impact of procedures directed at purging the graft of tumor cells will have to be determined in the adjuvant setting.

Negative purging has been tested in patients with BM metastases. Pharmacologic purging achieved a mean 2.5-log tumor-cell depletion, with marked engraftment delay.[126] Studies using immunomagnetic purging (IMP) showed a mean 3-log depletion of cancer cells, with no prolongation of the engraftment times compared to historical controls.[127] Both procedures combined resulted in a 4.5-log tumor-cell depletion,[128] at the expense of substantial engraftment delays.[129]

Positive selection targets the CD34 antigen, expressed on 0.5-3% of normal BM cells and PBPCs, including both the committed and, probably, the long-term reconstituting progenitor cells. The CD34 antigen does not appear to be expressed on breast cancer cells.[130] The University of Colorado BMTP reported a series of 155 breast cancer patients who received HDCT and a CD34-selected BM or PBPC graft.[131] CD34-selected stem cells effectively reconstituted immediate and long-term hematopoiesis. An average 2-log tumor-cell depletion was achieved. Patients receiving CD34+ PBPCs experienced neutrophil and platelet recovery rates that were comparable to patients who received unmanipulated grafts. Long-term follow-up showed that the durability of engraftment, immune reconstitution, DFS and OS, were comparable to patients receiving unmanipulated hematopoietic cell fractions.[132]

Since most patients still had detectable cancer cells present in their stem cell grafts following CD34-selection, maximally effective purging may require a combination of positive and negative-selection procedures. Preclinical studies have demonstrated a larger magnitude of tumor cell depletion using a sequential than with a simultaneous combination (averages 6.38-log and 4.29-log, respectively).[133] Patients receiving PBPCs purged with simultaneous CD34-selection and IMP experienced prompt and sustained engraftment.[134] Sequential positive and negative purging of PBPCs is presently under clinical evaluation. If it does not produce engraftment delays, a randomized trial will compare this approach to unmanipulated ASCT in patients with 10+ nodes receiving HDCT.

Other Lines of Future Progress

Clinical trials of allogeneic stem-cell transplantation are presently exploring a potential graft-versus-tumor (GVT) effect for breast cancer. Ueno et al. conducted a pilot study of this approach, and reported that a GVT effect may occur in breast cancer.[135] This needs to be confirmed in larger studies, and it is unclear whether the potential benefit will justify the risks of allogeneic transplantation.

Pursuing further a GVT effect, a "minitransplant" strategy is under evaluation at several institutions, using nonmyeloablative immunosuppressive preparative regimens that allow engraftment of allogeneic stem cells, as shown in patients with lymphoid malignancies.[136]

Dendritic cells are professional antigen presenting cells with high capacity to initiate the immune response.[137] Dendritic cells can be cultured from PBPCs and subsequently pulsed with a breast cancer antigen. Its use in the posttransplant setting against minimal residual disease holds promise.

Radioimmunotherapy, using ^{131}I-labeled-antiCD20, is highly active in B-cell lymphoma.[138,139,140] Its dose-limiting toxicity is myelosuppression. Stem cell-supported delivery of [90]Yttrium, conjugated to humanized BrE-3 monoclonal antibody, is presently being investigated for MBC. Preliminary results of a phase I PBPC-supported trial suggest the feasibility of a substantial dose-escalation of this isotope.[141]

The Her2/*neu* oncogene is overexpressed in 25%-30% of breast cancer patients.[142] Monoclonal antibodies against this oncogene (trastuzumab) have shown some activity in Her2/neu (+) tumors,[143] and in vitro synergy with cisplatin, carboplatin, docetaxel, etoposide and thiotepa.[144] Clinical studies of trastuzumab combined with chemotherapy, using cisplatin,[145] doxorubicin-cyclophosphamide[146] or paclitaxel,[119] showed an improved outcome compared with chemotherapy alone. Future trials will test the combination of trastuzumab with HDCT for Her2/neu (+) tumors.

CONCLUSIONS

High-dose chemotherapy constitutes an approach to improve results in breast cancer, based on a solid rationale. While initial phase II data are encouraging (Table 3), an answer to the important question of its relative merit over standard chemotherapy will only come from adequate phase III studies, and is still pending in most cases. In the meantime, it is imperative that research be continued, to improve HDCT combinations and to integrate them with novel therapies with different mechanisms of action.

Table 1. Classical Myeloablative Regimens

REGIMEN	COMPOSITION	AUTHOR
STAMP-I (CCB or CPB)	Cyclophosphamide 5625 mg/m^2 Cisplatin 165 mg/m^2 BCNU 600 mg m^2	Peters et al [24]
STAMP-V (CTCb)	Cyclophosphamide 6000 mg/m^2 Thiotepa 500 mg/m^2 Carboplatin 800 mg/m^2	Eder et al [26]
CT	Cyclophosphamide 7500 mg/m^2 Thiotepa 675 mg/m^2	Williams et al [27]

Table 2. Sequential Strategies on HDC for MBC

STRATEGY	REGIMEN	# Pts	% CR	% Long-term DFS
Refractory disease	STAMP-I [24] STAMP-V [26]	23 16	26 6	0 0
Upfront treatment for MBC	STAMP-I [28]	22	54	14
Consolidation after induction	AFM ➔ STAMP-I [29] AFM ➔ STAMP-V [30] LOMAC/ FCAP ➔ CT [31]	45 29 62	57 45 32	22 (&), 26 (†) 17 13 (&), 17 (†)

(&) DFS based on an intent-to-treat analyses.
(†) DFS for patients actually treated with HDC.

Table 3. Overall Results from the Major Phase II Trials of HDC for Breast Cancer

SETTING	Long-term DFS	Reference
4-9 nodes	>70 %	94, 95, 96
10+ nodes	56% to 65 %	91, 92
Inflammatory carcinoma	70 %	100, 101
Metastatic chemosensitive disease	15% to 25 %	29, 30, 31
Metastatic with no evidence of disease (NED)	55%	40

Figure 1. Randomized Trials for Metastatic Breast Cancer in Both Trials

Figure 1A. Duke/CALGB Study

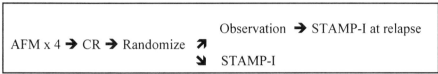

AFM: doxorubicin - 5-fluorouracil- methotrexate. CR: complete remission.
STAMP-I: high-dose cyclophosphamide- cisplatin-BCNU.

Figure 1B. Philadelphia/ECOG Study

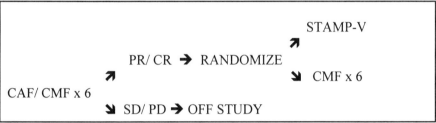

CAF: cyclophosphamide, doxorubicin and 5-fluorouracil; CMF:
cyclophosphamide, methotrexate and 5-fluorouracil; PR: partial response; CR:
complete response; SD: stable disease; PD: progressive disease; STAMP-V:
high-dose cyclophosphamide, thiotepa and carboplatin.

Figure 1C. South African Trial

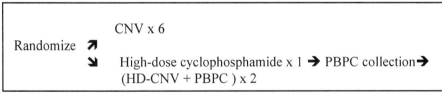

CNV: cyclophosphamide-mitoxantrone-vincristine; PBPC: peripheral blood
progenitor cells; HD-CNV: high-dose cyclophosphamide-mitoxantrone-
etoposide

Figure 2. Randomized Trials for Breast Cancer Patients with 10+ Nodes

Figure 2A. Intergroup Trial (CALGB / SWOG / NCIC)

```
                            CAF x 1 ➜ STAMP-I ➜ XRT + Tamoxifen
CAF x 3 ➜ Randomize ➚
                        ➘ CAF x 1 ➜ intermediate-dose CCB ➜ XRT
                            + Tamoxifen
```

CALGB: Cancer and Leukemia Group B; SWOG: Southwestern Oncology Group; NCIC: National Institute of Cancer of Canada; CAF: standard-dose cyclophosphamide-doxorubicin-5-fluorouracil. STAMP-I: high-dose CCB (cyclophosphamide- cisplatin-BCNU). XRT: radiotherapy.

Figure 2B. ECOG Trial

```
                    CAF x 6 ➜ HD CPA-TT ➜ XRT + Tamoxifen
Randomize ➚
          ➘    CAF x 6 ➜ XRT + Tamoxifen
```

ECOG: Eastern Cooperative Oncology Group; HD CPA-TT: high-dose cyclophosphamide-thiotepa

Figure 2C. South African Trial

```
                CAF x 6
Randomize ➚
          ➘    High-dose cyclophosphamide x 1 ➜
                PBPC collection ➜ (HD-CNV + PBPC ) x 2
```

CAF: cyclophosphamide-doxorubicin-fluorouracil; PBPC: peripheral blood progenitor cells; HD-CNV: high-dose cyclophosphamide-mitoxantrone-etoposide

Figure 3. Intergroup Randomized Trial for Patients with 4-9 Nodes

```
+-------------------------------------------------------------------+
|                    AC x 4 ➔ STAMP-I / STAMP-V  ➔ XRT + Tamoxifen   |
|      Randomize ➚                                                    |
|                ➘  (AAA - TTT -  CCC) + G-CSF   ➔  XRT + Tamoxifen  |
+-------------------------------------------------------------------+
```

AC: standard-dose doxorubicin-cyclophosphamide. STAMP-I: high-dose
cyclophosphamide- cisplatin-BCNU. STAMP-V: high-dose cyclophosphamide-
thiotepa-carboplatin. AAA: doxorubicin x 3. TTT: Taxol x 3. CCC:
cyclophosphamide x 3.

Figure 4. Relapse-free survival (RFS) and overall survival (OS) of metastatic breast cancer patients with no evidence of disease (NED) (University of Colorado BMTP)

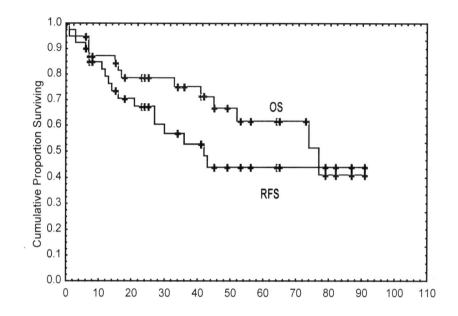

Figure 5. Relapse-free survival (RFS) and overall survival for inflammatory breast carcinoma (University of Colorado BMTP)

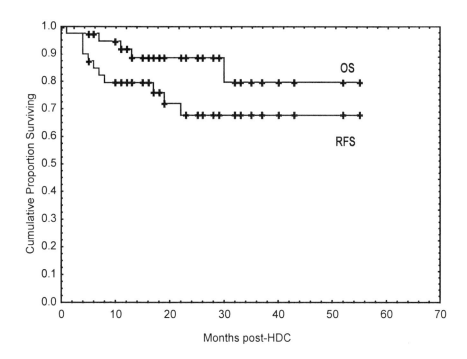

Figure 6. Relapse-free survival curves of high-risk primary breast cancer patients treated at the University of Colorado BMT Program, stratified according to the Colorado model

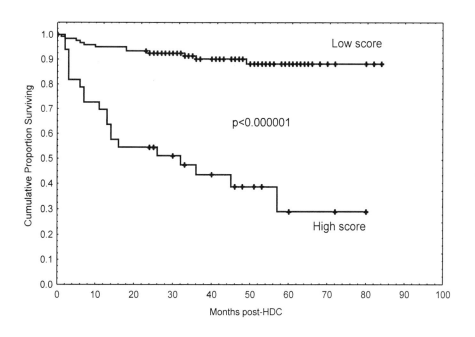

REFERENCES:

1. Peters WP, Henner WD, Bast RC, Schnipper L, Frei III E. Novel toxicities associated with high dose combination alkylating agents in autologous bone marrow support. In Dicke KA, Spitzer G, Zander AR (eds): Autologous Bone Marrow Transplantation: Proceedings of the First International Symposium. University of Texas Cancer center, MD Anderson Hospital, Houston, pp 231-235, 1986.

2. Antman KH, Rowlings PA, Vaughan WP, et al. High-dose chemotherapy with autologous hematopoietic stem-cell support for breast cancer in North America. J Clin Oncol 15: 1870-1879, 1997.

3. Hryniuk W, Busch H. The importance of dose intensity in chemotherapy of metastatic breast cancer. J Clin Oncol 2: 1281-1288, 1984.

4. Hryniuk W, Frei III E, Wright FA. A single scale for comparing dose-intensity of all chemotherapy regimens in breast cancer: Summation dose-intensity. J Clin Oncol 16: 3137-3147, 1998.

5. Hryniuk W, Levine MN. Analysis of dose intensity for adjuvant chemotherapy trials in stage II breast cancer. J Clin Oncol 4: 1162-1170, 1986.

6. Bonadonna G, Valagussa P. Dose-response effect of adjuvant chemotherapy in breast cancer. N Eng J Med 304: 10-15, 1981.

7. Tannock IF, Boyd NF, DeBoer G, et al. A randomized trial of two doses of cyclophosphamide, methotrexate and fluorouracil for patients with metastatic breast cancer. J Clin Oncol 6: 1377-1387, 1988.

8. Hortobagyi GN, Bodey GP, Buzdar AU, et al. Evaluation of high-dose versus standard FAC chemotherapy for advanced breast cancer in protected environment units: A prospective randomized study. J Clin Oncol 5: 354-364, 1987.

9. Winer E. Berry D, Duggan D, et al. Failure of higher dose paclitaxel to improve outcome in aptients with metastatic breast cancer - Results from CALGB 9342. Proc Am Soc Clin Oncol 1998; 17:101a.

10. Habeshaw T, Paul R, Jones R, et al. Epirubicin at two dose levels with prednisolone as treatment for advanced breast cancer: The results of a randomized trial. J Clin Oncol 9: 295-304, 1991.

11. Bastholt L, Dalmark M, Gjedde SB, et al. Dose-response relationship of epirubicin in the treatment of postmenopausal patients with metastatic breast cancer: A randomized study of epirubicin at four different dose levels

performed by the Danish Breast Cancer Cooperative Group. J Clin Oncol 1996; 14:1146-1155.

12.   Brufman G, Corajort E, Ghilezan N, et al. Doubling epirubicin dose intensity (100 mg/m^2 versus 50 mg/m^2) in the FEC regimen significantly increases response rate. An international randomized phase III study in metastatic breast cancer. Ann Oncol 1997; 8:155-162.

13.   Focan C, Andrien JM, Closon Mth, et al. Dose-response relationship of epirubicin based first-line chemotherapy for advanced breast cancer: A prospective randomized trial. J Clin Oncol 1993; 11:1253-1263.

14.   Fountzilas G, Athanassiades A, Giannakkais T, et al. A randomized study of epirubicin monotherapy every four or every two weeks in advanced breast cancer. A Hellenic Cooperative Oncology Group study. Ann Oncol 1997; 8:1213-1220.

15.   Wood WC, Budman DR, Korzun AH, et al. Dose and dose intensity of adjuvant chemotherapy for stage II, node-positive breast carcinoma. N Eng J Med 330: 1253-1259, 1994.

16.   Budman DR, Berry DA, Cirrincione CT, et al. Dose and dose intensity as determinants of outcome in the adjuvant treatment of breast cancer. J Natl Cancer Inst 91: 286-287, 1999.

17.   Bonneterre J, Roché H, Bremond A, et al. Results of a randomized trial of adjuvant chemotherapy with FEC 50 vs. FEC 100 in high risk node-positive breast cancer patients. Proc Am Soc Clin Oncol 17: 124a, 1998.

18.   Fisher B, Anderson S, Wickerham S, et al. Increased intensification and total dose of cyclophosphamide in a doxorubicin-cyclophosphamide regimen for the treatment of primary breast cancer: Findings from National Surgical Adjuvant Breast and Bowel Project B-22. J Clin Oncol 15: 1858-1869, 1997.

19.   Wolmark N, Fisher B, Anderson S. The effect of increasing dose intensity and cumulative dose of adjuvant cyclophosphamide in node positive breast cancer: Results of NSABP B-25. Breast Cancer Res Treat 46 (1): 26, 1997.

20.   Henderson IC, Berry D, Demetri G, et al. Improved disease-free and overall survival from the addition of sequential paclitaxel but not from the escalation of doxorubicin dose level in the adjuvant chemotherapy of patients with node-positive primary breast cancer. Proc Am Soc Clin Oncol 17:101a, 1998.

21.   Greenberg PA, Hortobagyi GN, Smith TL, et al. Long-term follow-up of patients with complete remission following combination chemotherapy for metastatic breast cancer. J Clin Oncol 14: 2197-2205, 1996.

22. Frei III E, Canellos GP. Dose: A critical factor in cancer chemotherapy. Amer J Med 69: 585-594, 1980.

23. Frei III E, Antman K, Teicher B, Eder P,et al. Bone Marrow Autotransplantation for solid tumors - Prospects. J Clin Oncol 4: 515-526, 1989.

24. Peters WP, Eder JP, Henner WD, et al. High-dose combination chemotherapy with autologous bone marrow support: A phase I trial. J Clin Oncol 4: 646-654, 1986.

25. Eder JP, Antman K, Peters WP, et al. High dose combination alkylating agent chemotherapy with autologous bone marrow support for metastatic breast cancer. J Clin Oncol 4: 646-654, 1986.

26. Eder JP, Elias A, Shea TC, et al. A phase I-II study of cyclophosphamide, thiotepa, and carboplatin with autologous bone marrow transplantation in solid tumor patients. J Clin Oncol 8: 1239-1245, 1990.

27. Williams SF, Bitran JD, Kaminer L, et al. A phase I-II study of bialkylator chemotherapy, high-dose thiotepa, and cyclophosphamide with autologous bone marrow reinfusion in patients with advanced cancer. J Clin Oncol 5: 260-265, 1990.

28. Peters WP, Shpall EJ, Jones RB, et al. High-dose combination chemotherapy with bone marrow support as initial treatment for metastatic breast cancer. J Clin Oncol 6: 1368-1376, 1988.

29. Jones RB, Shpall EJ, Ross M, et al. AFM induction chemotherapy followed by intensive alkylating agent consolidation with autologous bone marrow support (ABMS) for advanced breast cancer: current results. Proc Am Soc Clin Oncol 7: 121, 1990.

30. Antman K, Ayash L, Elias A, et al. A phase II study of high-dose cyclophosphamide, thiotepa, and carboplatin with autologous bone marrow support in women with measurable advanced breast cancer responding to standard-dose therapy. J Clin Oncol 10: 102-110, 1992.

31. Williams SF, Gilewski T, Mick R, et al. High-dose consolidation therapy with autologous stem cell rescue in stage IV breast cancer: Follow-up report. J Clin Oncol 10: 1743-1747, 1992.

32. Jones RB, Shpall EJ, Shogan J, et al. The Duke AFM program. Intensive induction chemotherapy for metastatic breast cancer. Cancer 66: 431-436, 1990.

33. Decker DA, Ahman DL, Bisel HF, et al. Complete responders to

chemotherapy in metastatic breast cancer. Characterization and analysis. JAMA 242: 2075-2079, 1979.

34. Powles TJ, Smith IE, Ford HT, et al. Failure of chemotherapy to prolong survival in a group of patients with metastatic breast cancer. Lancet 1:580-582, 1980.

35. Smith GA, Henderson IC. High-dose chemotherapy (HDC) with autologous bone marrow transplantation (ABMT) for the treatment of breast cancer: The jury is still out. In Hellman S, and Rosenberg SA (eds), pp 201-214, 1995.

36. Rahman ZU, Frye DK, Buzdar AU, et al. Impact of selection process on response rate and long-term survival of potential high-dose chemotherapy candidates treated with standard-dose doxorubicin-containing chemotherapy in patients with metastatic breast cancer. J Clin Oncol 15:3171-3177, 1997.

37. Dunphy FR, Spitzer G, Rossiter JE, et al. Factors predicting long-term survival for metastatic breast cancer patients treated with high-dose chemotherapy and bone marrow support. Cancer 73: 2157-2167, 1994.

38. Ayash LJ, Wheeler C, Fairclough D, et al. Prognostic factors for prolonged progression-free survival with high-dose chemotherapy with autologous stem-cell support for advanced breast cancer. J Clin Oncol 13: 2043-2049, 1995.

39. Doroshow JH, Somlo G, Ahn C, et al. Prognostic factors predicting progression-free and overall survival in patients with responsive metastatic breast cancer treated with high-dose chemotherapy and bone marrow stem cell reinfusion. Proc Am Soc Clin Oncol 14: 319a, 1995.

40. Nieto Y, Cagnoni PJ, Shpall EJ, et al. Prospective phase II study of high-dose chemotherapy with autologous stem cell transplant for patients with stage IV breast cancer with minimal metastases. Clin Cancer Res 5: 1731-1737, 1999.

41. Laport GF, Grad G, Grinblatt DL, et al. High-dose chemotherapy consolidation with autologous stem cell rescue in metastatic breast cancer: A 10-year experience. Bone Marrow Transplant 21: 127-132, 1998.

42. Sledge GW, Loehrer PJ, Roht BJ, Einhorn LH. Cisplatin as first-line therapy for metastatic breats cancer. J Clin Oncol 6: 1811-1814, 1988.

43. Martín M, Díaz-Rubio E, Casado A, et al. Carboplatin: An active drug in metastatic breast cancer. J Clin Oncol 10: 433-437, 1992.

44. Tew K, Colvin OM, Chabner BA. Alkylating agents. In: BA Chabner and DL Longo (eds), Cancer Chemotherapy and Biotherapy, 2nd edition, pp 297-332. Philadelphia: Lippincott-Raven, 1996.

45. Chen T-L, Passos-Coelho JL, Noe DA, et al. Nonlinear pharmacokinetics of cyclophosphamide in patients with metastatic breast cancer receiving high-dose chemotherapy followed by autologous bone marrow transplantation. Cancer Res 55: 810-816, 1996.

46. Nieto Y, Xu X, Cagnoni PJ, et al. Nonpredictable pharmacokinetic behavior of high-dose cyclophosphamide in combination with cisplatin and 1,3-bis(2-chloroethyl)-1-nitrosourea. Clin Cancer Res 5: 747-751, 1999.

47. Busse D, Busch FW, Bohnenstengel F, Eichelbaum M, Fischer P, Opalinska J, Schumacher K, Schweizer E, Kroemer HK. Dose escalation of cyclophosphamide in patients with breast cancer: Consequences for pharmacokinetics and metabolism. J Clin Oncol 15: 1885-1896, 1997.

48. Doroshow JH. Anthracyclines and anthracenediones. In: Chabner BA and Longo DL (eds). Cancer Chemotherapy and Biotherapy. Lippincott-Raven, 2nd ed., 1996.

49. Eisenhauer EA, Ten Bokkel Huinink WW, Swenerton KD, et al. European-Canadian randomized trial of paclitaxel in relapsed ovarian cancer: High-dose versus low-dose and long versus short infusion. J Clin Oncol 12: 2654-2666, 1994.

50. Kohn EC, Sarosy G, Bicher A, et al. Dose intense taxol: High response rate in patients with platinum resistant recurrent ovarian cancer. J Natl Cancer Inst 86:18-24, 1994.

51. Raymond E, Hanauske A, Faivre S, Izbicka E, Clark G, Rowinsky EK, Von Hoff DD. Effects of prolonged versus short-term exposure paclitaxel on human tumor colony-forming units. Anticancer Drugs 8: 379-385, 1997.

52. Hanauske AR, Degen D, Hilsenbeck SG, et al. Effects of Taxotere and Taxol in vitro colony formation of freshly explanted human tumour cells. Anticancer Drugs 3: 121-124, 1992.

53. García P, Braguer D, Carkes G, et al. Comparative effects of taxol and taxotere on two different human carcinoma cell lines. Cancer Chemother Pharmacol 34: 335-343, 1994.

54. Donehower RC, Rowinsky EK, Grochow LB,et al. Phase I trial of taxol in patients with advanced cancer. Cancer Treatment Rep 71: 1171-1177, 1987.

55. Aapro MS, Zulian G, Alberto P, et al. Phase I and pharmacokinetic study of RP 569876 in a new ethanol-free formulation of Taxotere. Ann Oncol 3 (Suppl 5): 208, 1992.

56. Extra JM, Rousseau F, Bruno R, et al. Phase I and pharmacokinetic study of

Taxotere (RP 569876; NSC 628503) given as a short intravenous infusion. Cancer Res 53: 1037-1042, 1993.

57.   Stemmer SM, Cagnoni PJ, Shpall EJ, et al. High-dose paclitaxel, cyclophosphamide, and cisplatin with autologous hematopoietic progenitor-cell support: A phase I trial. J Clin Oncol 14: 1463-1472, 1996.

58.   Mamounas E, Brown A, Smith R, et al. Effect of taxol duration of infusion in advanced breast cancer (ABC): Results from NSABP-26 trial comparing 2- to 24-hr infusion of high-dose taxol. Proc Am Soc Clin Oncol 17: 101a, 1998.

59.   Omura GA, Brady MF, Delmore JE, et al. A randomized trial of paclitaxel at 2 dose levels and filgastrim (G-CSF) at 2 doses in platinum pretreated epithelial ovarian cancer: a Gynecologic Oncology Group, SWOG, NCTTG and ECOG study. Proc Am Soc Clin Oncol 15: 280a, 1996.

60.   Bonomi P, Kim K, Chang A, Johnson D. Phase III trial comparing etoposide-cisplatin versus taxol with cisplatin-G-CSF versus taxol-cisplatin in advanced non-small cell lung cancer. An Eastern Cooperative Oncology Group (ECOG) trial. Proc Am Soc Clin Oncol 15: 382a, 1996.

61.   Fields KK, Elfenbein GJ, Perkins JB, et al. High versus standard dose chemotherapy for the treatment of breast cancer. Annals New York Academy of Sciences 770: 288-304, 1995.

62.   Mayordomo JI, Yubero A, Cajal R, et al. Phase I trial of high-dose paclitaxel in combination with cyclophosphamide, thiotepa and carboplatin with autologous peripheral blood stem cell rescue. Proc Am Soc Clin Oncol 16: 102a, 1997.

63.   Chan S, Friedrichs K, Noel D, et al. A phase III study of taxotere7 vs. doxorubicin in patients with metastatic breast cancer who have failed an alkylating containing regimen. Breast Cancer Res Treat 46 (1): 23, 1997.

64.   Valero V. Docetaxel as single-agent therapy in metastatic breast cancer: Clinical efficacy. Semin Oncol 24 (4, suppl 13): S13-11-S13-18, 1997.

65.   Valero V, Holmes FA, Walters RS, et al. Phase II study of docetaxel: A new, highly effective antineoplastic agent in the management of patients with anthracycline-resistant metastatic breast cancer. J Clin Oncol 13: 2886-2894, 1995.

66.   Ravdin PM, Burris HA III, Cook G, et al. Phase II trial of docetaxel in advanced anthracycline-resistant or anthracenedione-resistant breast cancer. J Clin Oncol 13: 2879-2885, 1995.

67. Dunphy FR, Spitzer G, Buzdar AU, et al: Treatment of estrogen receptor-negative or hormonally refractory breast cancer with double high-dose chemotherapy intensification and bone marrow support. J Clin Oncol 8: 1207-1216, 1990.

68. Crown J, Kritz A, Vahdat K, et al. Rapid administration of multiple cycles of high-dose myelosuppressive chemotherapy in patients with metastatic breast cancer. J Clin Oncol 11: 1144-1149, 1993.

69. Shapiro CL, Ayash L, Webb IJ, et al. Repetitive cycles of cyclophosphamide, thiotepa, and carboplatin intensification with peripheral-blood progenitor cells and filgrastim in advanced breast cancer patients. J Clin Oncol 15: 674-683, 1997.

70. Ayash LJ, Elias A, Wheeler C, et al. Double dose-intensive chemotherapy with autologous marrow and peripheral-blood progenitor-cell support for metastatic breast cancer: A feasibility study. J Clin Oncol 12: 37-44, 1994.

71. Rodenhuis S, Westermann A, Holtkamp MJ, et al. Feasibility of multiple courses of high-dose cyclophosphamide, thiotepa, and carboplatin for breast cancer or germ cell cancer. J Clin Oncol 14: 1473-1483, 1996.

72. Broun ER, Sridhara R, Sledge GW, et al. Tandem autotransplantion for the treatment of metastatic breast cancer. J Clin Oncol 13: 2050-2055, 1995.

73. Ayash LJ, Elias A, Schwartz G, et al. Double dose-intensive chemotherapy with autologous stem-cell support for metastatic breast cancer: No improvement in progression-free survival by the sequence of high-dose melphalan followed by cyclophosphamide, thiotepa, and carboplatin. J Clin Oncol 14: 2984-2992, 1996.

74. Bitran JD, Samuels B, Klein L, et al. Tandem high-dose chemotherapy supported by hematopoietic progenitor cells yields prolonged survival in stage IV breast cancer. Bone Marrow Transplant 17: 157-162, 1996.

75. Teicher BA, Ara G, Keyes SR, et al. Acute in vivo resistance in high-dose therapy. Clin Cancer Res 4: 483-491, 1998.

76. Bezwoda WR, Seymour L, Dansey RD. High-dose chemotherapy with hematopoietic rescue as primary treatment for metastatic breast cancer: A randomized trial. J Clin Oncol 13: 2483-2489, 1995.

77. Bezwoda WR. Primary high dose chemotherapy for metastatic breast cancer: Update and analysis of prognostic factors. Proc Am Soc Clin Oncol 17: 115a, 1998.

78.   Bezwoda WR, Seymour L, Ariad S. First line chemotherapy of advanced breast cancer with mitoxantrone, cyclophosphamide and vincristine. Oncology 46: 208-211, 1989.

79.   Sparano JA, Hu P, Rao RM, et al. Phase II trial of doxorubicin plus paclitaxel plus G-CSF in metastatic breast cancer (MBC): An Eastern Oncology Cooperative Group study (E4195. Breast Cancer Res Treat 46: 23a, 1997.

80.   Irwin LE, Chlebowski RT. Weiner JM, et al. Randomized comparinson of two combination chemotherapy regimens containing doxorubicin in patients with metastatic breast cancer: a Western Cancer Study Group Trial. Cancer Treat Rep 64: 981-984, 1980.

81.   Tranum BL, McDonald B, Thigpen T, et al. Adriamycin combinations in advanced breast cancer. A Southwest Oncology Group study. Cancer 49: 835-839, 1982.

82.   Kennealey GT, Boston B, Mitchell MS, et al. Combination chemotherapy for advanced breast cancer: two regimens containing adriamycin. Cancer 42: 27-33, 1978.

83.   Sparano JA, Speyer J, Gradishar WJ, et al. Phase I trial of escalating doses of paclitaxel plus doxorubicin and dexrazoxane in patients with advanced breast cancer. J Clin Oncol 17: 880-886, 1999.

84.   Peters WP, Jones RB, Vredenburgh J, et al. A large, prospective, randomized trial of high-dose combination alkylating agents (CPB) with autologous cellular support (ABMS) as consolidation for patients with metastatic breast cancer achieving complete remission after intensive doxorubicin-based induction therapy (AFM). Proc Am Soc Clin Oncol 15: 121a, 1996.

85.   Stadtmauer EA, O'Neill A, Godstein LJ, et al. Phase III randomized trial of high-dose chemotherapy (HDC) and stem cell support (SCT) shows no difference in overall survival or severe toxicity compared to maintenance chemotherapy with cyclophosphamide, methotrexate and 5-fluorouracil (CMF) for women with metastatic breast cancer who are responding to conventional induction chemotherapy: The "Philadelphia" Intergroup study (PBT-1). Proc Am Soc Clin Oncol 18: 1a, 1999.

86.   Lotz J-P, Curé H, Janvier M, et al. High-dose chemotherapy (HD-CT) with hematopoietic stem cells transplantation (HSCT) for metastatic breast cancer (MBC): Results of the French Protocol PEGASE 04. Proc Am Soc Clin Oncol 18: 43a, 1999.

87.   Bonadonna G, Valagussa P. Adjuvant systemic therapy for resectable breast

cancer. J Clin Oncol 3: 259-275, 1985.
88. Bonadonna G, Zambetti M, Valagussa P. Sequential or alternating doxorubicin and CMF regimens in breast cancer with more than three positive nodes. Ten-year results. JAMA 273: 542-547, 1995.
89. Hryniuk W, Levine MN. Analysis of dose intensity for adjuvant chemotherapy trials in stage II breast cancer. J Clin Oncol 4: 1162-1170, 1986.
90. Peters WP, Ross M, Vredenburgh JJ, et al. High-dose chemotherapy and autologous bone marrow suppport as consolidation after standard-dose adjuvant therapy for high-risk primary breast cancer. J Clin Oncol 11: 1132-1143, 1993.
91. Peters WP. Berry D, Vredenburgh JJ, et al. Five year follow-up of high-dose combination alkylating agents with ABMT as consolidation after standard-dose CAF for primary breast cancer involving ∃10 axillary lymph nodes (Duke/CALGB 8782). Proc Am Soc Clin Oncol 14: 317a, 1995.
92. Gianni AM, Siena S, Bregni M, et al. Efficacy, toxicity and applicability of high-dose chemotherapy as adjuvant treatment in operable breast cancer with 10 or more involved axillary nodes: Five-year results. J Clin Oncol 15: 2312-2321, 1997.
93. Buzzoni R, Bonadonna G, Valagussa P, et al. Adjuvant chemotherapy with doxorubicin plus cyclophosphamide, methotrexate and fluorouracil in the treatment of resectable breast cancer with more than three positive nodes. J Clin Oncol 9: 2134-2140, 1991.
94. Bearman SI, Overmoyer BA, Bolwell BJ, et al. High-dose chemotherapy with autologous peripheral blood progenitor cell support for primary breast cancer in patients with 4-9 involved axillary lymph nodes. Bone Marrow Transplantation 20: 931-937, 1997.
95. Hussein A, Plummer M, Vredenburgh J, et al. High-dose chemotherapy (HDC) with cyclophosphamide, cisplatin, and BCNU (CPB) and autologous bone marrow and peripheral blood progenitor cells for stage II/III breast cancer involving 4-9 axillary lymph nodes. Proc Am Soc Clin Oncol 15: 350a, 1996.
96. De Graaf H, Willemse PHB, De Vries EGE, et al. Intensive chemotherapy with autologous bone marrow transfusion as primary treatment in women with breast cancer and more than five involved axillary lymph nodes. Eur J Cancer 30A, 150-153, 1994.

97. Hudis C, Seidman A, Baselga J, et al. Sequential dose-dense doxorubicin, paclitaxel, and cyclophosphamide for resectable high-risk breast cancer: Feasibility and efficacy. J Clin Oncol 17: 93-100, 1999.

98. Jaiyesimi IA, Buzdar AU, Hortobagyi G. Inflammatory breast cancer: A review. J Clin Oncol 10: 1014-1024, 1992.

99. Thomas F, Arriagada R, Spielmann M, et al. Pattern of failure in patients with inflammatory breast cancer treated by alternating radiotherapy and chemotherapy. Cancer 76: 2286-2290, 1995.

100. Ayash L, Elias A, Ibrahim J, et al. High-dose multimodality therapy with autologous stem cell support for stage IIIB breast cancer. J Clin Oncol 16: 1000-1007, 1998.

101. Cagnoni PJ, Nieto Y, Shpall EJ, et al. High-dose chemotherapy with autologous progenitor cell support as part of combined modality therapy for inflammatory breast cancer. J Clin Oncol 16: 1661-1668, 1998.

102. Nieto Y, Cagnoni PJ, Shpall EJ, et al. Predictive model for relapse after high-dose chemotherapy with peripheral blood progenitor cell support for high-risk primary breast cancer. Clin Cancer Res 5:3425-3431, 1999.

103. Nieto Y, Nawaz S, Cagnoni PJ, et al. Overexpression of Her-2/neu (H2N), but not p53 mutations, is a poor prognostic factor in high-risk primary breast cancer (HRPBC) treated with high-dose chemotherapy (HDC) and autologous stem-cell transplant (ASCT). Proc Am Soc Clin Oncol 18: 77a, 1999.

104. Somlo G, Doroshow JH, Forman SJ, et al. High-dose chemotherapy and stem-cell rescue in the treatment of high-risk breast cancer: Prognostic indicators of progression-free and overall survival. J Clin Oncol 15: 2882-2893, 1997.

105. Crump M, Goss PE, Prince M, et al. Outcome of extensive evaluation before adjuvant therapy in women with breast cancer and ten or more positive axillary lymph nodes. J Clin Oncol 14: 66-69, 1996.

106. García-Carbonero R, Hidalgo M, Paz-Ares L, et al. Patient selection in high-dose chemotherapy trials: Relevance in high-risk breast cancer. J Clin Oncol 15: 3178-3184, 1997.

107. Rodenhuis S, Richel DJ, van der Wall E, et al. Randomised trial of high-dose chemotherapy and haempopoietic progenitor-cell support in operable breast cancer with extensive axillary involvement. Lancet 352: 515-521, 1998.

108. Hortobagyi GN, Buzdar AU, Champlin R, et al. Lack of efficacy of adjuvant

high-dose tandem combination chemotherapy for high-risk primary breast cancer - A randomized trial. Proc Am Soc Clin Oncol 17: 123a, 1998.

109. Dunphy FR, Spitzer G, Buzdar AU, et al. Treatment of estrogen receptor-negative or hormonally refractory breast cancer with double high-dose chemotherapy intensification and bone marrow support. J Clin Oncol 8: 1207-1216, 1990.

110. Neidhart JE, Kohler W, Stidley C, et al. A phase I study of repeated cycles of high-dose cyclophosphamide, etoposide and cisplatin administered without bone marrow transplantation. J Clin Oncol 8: 1728-1738, 1990.

111. Peters WP, Rosner G, Vredenburgh J, et al. A prospective, randomized comparison of two doses of combination alkylating agents as consolidation after CAF in high-risk primary breast cancer involving ten or more axillary lymph nodes: Preliminary results of CALGB 9082/SWOG 9114/NCIC MA-13. Proc Am Soc Clin Oncol 18: 1a, 1999.

112. Bezwoda WR. Randomised, controlled trial of high dose chemotherapy (HD-CNVp) versus standard dose (CAF) chemotherapy for high risk, surgically treated, primary breast cancer. Proc Am Soc Clin Oncol 18: 2a, 1999.

113. The Scandinavian Study Group 9401. Results from a randomized adjuvant breast cancer study with high dose chemotherapy with CTCb supported by autologous bone marrow stem cells versus dose escalated and tailored FEC therapy. Proc Am Soc Clin Oncol 18: 2a, 1999.

114. Philip T, Chauvin F, Bron D, et al. PARMA international protocol: Pilot study on 50 patients and preliminary analysis of the ongoing randomized study (62 patients). Ann Oncol 2: 57-64 (Suppl), 1991.

115. Bron D, Philip T, Guglielmi C, et al. The PARMA international randomized study in relpased non-Hodgkin's lymphoma. Analysis on the first 153 preincluded patients. Exp Hematol 19 (6):546, 1991.

116. Philip T, Guglielmi C, Hagenbeek A, et al. Autologous bone marrow transplantation as compared with salvage chemotherapy in relapses of chemotherapy-sensitive non-Hodgkins's lymphoma. N Engl J Med 333: 1540-1545, 1995.

117. Ross AA, Cooper BW, Lazarus HM, et al: Detection and viability of tumor cells in peripheral blood stem cell collections from breast cancer patients using immunocytochemical and clonogenic assay techniques. Blood 82: 2605, 1993.

118. Schoenfeld A, Kruger KH, Gomm J, et al. The detection of micrometastases

in the peripheral blood and bone marrow of patients with breast cancer using immunohistochemistry and reverse transcriptase polymerase chain reaction for keratin 19. Eur J Cancer 33: 854-861, 1997.

119. Datta YH, Adams PT, Drobyski WR, Ethier SP, Terry VH, Roth MS. Sensitive detection of occult breast cancer by the reverse-transcriptase polymerase chain reaction. J Clin Oncol 12: 475-482, 1994.

120. Fields KK, Elfenbein GJ, Trudeau WL. Clinical significance of bone marrow metastases in patients with breast cancer undergoing high-dose chemotherapy and autologous bone marrow transplantation. J Clin Oncol 14: 1868-1876, 1996.

121. Franklin W, Shpall EJ, Archer P, et al: Immunocytochemical detection of breast cancer cells in marrow and peripheral blood of patients undergoing high dose chemotherapy with autologous stem cell support. Breast Cancer Res Treat 41: 1-13, 1996.

122. Sharp JC, Kessinger A, Mann S, et al: Detection and clinical significance of minimal tumor cell contamination of peripheral blood stem cell harvests. Int J Cell Clon 10 (suppl 1): 92-94, 1992.

123. Vredenburgh J, Silva O, Broadwater G, et al: The significance of tumor contamination in the bone marrow from high-risk primary breast cancer patients treated with high-dose chemotherapy and hematopoietic support. Biol Blood Marrow Transplant 3: 91-97, 1997.

124. Umiel T, Moss TJ, Cooper B, et al. The prognostic value of bone marrow micrometastases in stage II/III breast cancer patients undergoing autologous transplant (ABMT) therapy. Proc Am Soc Clin Oncol 17: 79a, (abstract #306), 1998.

125. Cooper BW, Moss TJ, Ross AA, Ybanez J, and Lazarus HM. Occult tumor contamination of hematopoietic stem-cell product does not affect clinical outcome of autologous transplantation in patients with metastatic breast cancer. J Clin Oncol 16: 3509-3517, 1998.

126. Shpall EJ, Jones RB, Bast RC, et al: 4-Hydroperoxycyclophosphamide purging of breast cancer from the mononuclear cell fraction of bone marrow in patients receiving high-dose chemotherapy and autologous marrow support: A phase I trial. J Clin Oncol 9: 85-93, 1991.

127. Shpall EJ, Bast RC, Joines WT, et al: Immunomagnetic purging of breast cancer from bone marrow for autologous transplantation. Bone Marrow Transplantation 7: 145-151, 1991.

128. Anderson IC, Shpall EJ, Leslie DS, et al. Elimination of malignant clonogenic breast cancer cells from human bone marrow. Cancer Res 15: 4659, 1989.

129. Vredenburgh JJ, Hussein A, Rubin P, et al: High-dose chemotherapy and immunomagnetically purged peripheral blood progenitor cells and bone marrow for metastatic breast carcinoma. Proc Am Soc Clin Oncol 15: 339, 1996 [Abstract #983].

130. Krause DS, Fackler MJ, Civin CI, and Stratford May W: CD34: Structure, biology and clinical utility. Blood 87: 1-13, 1996.

131. Shpall EJ, Jones RB, Bearman SI, et al: Transplantation of enriched CD34-positive autologous marrow into breast cancer patients following high-dose chemotherapy: Influence of CD34-positive peripheral-blood progenitors and growth factors on engraftment. J Clin Oncol 12: 28-36, 1994.

132. Shpall EJ, Bearman SI, Cagnoni PJ, et al. Long-term follow-up of CD34-positive hematopoietic progenitor cell support for breast cancer patients receiving high-dose chemotherapy. J Clin Oncol *(In press).*

133. University of Colorado, unpublished observations.

134. Mohr M, Hilgenfeld E, Fietz B, et al. Efficacy and safety of simultaneous immunomagnetic CD34+ cell selection and breast cancer cell purging in peripheral blood progenitor cell samples used for hematopoietic rescue after high-dose therapy. Clin Cancer Res 5: 1035-1040, 1999.

135. Ueno NT, Rondón G, Mirza NQ, et al. Allogeneic peripheral-blood progenitor-cell transplantation for poor-risk patients with metastatic breast cancer. J Clin Oncol 16: 986-993, 1998.

136. Khouri IF, Keating M, Körbling M, et al. Transplant-lite: Induction of graft-versus-malignancy using fludarabine-based nonablative chemotherapy and allogeneic blood progenitor-cell transplantation as treatment for lymphoid malignancies. J Clin Oncol 16: 2817-2824, 1998.

137. Steinman RM. The dendritic cell system and its role in immunogenicity. Ann Rev Immunol 9: 271-296, 1991.

138. Press O, Eary J, Appelbaum J, et al. Radiolabeled antibody therapy of B-cell lymphoma with autologous bone marrow support. N Engl J Med 329: 1219, 1993.

139. Kaminski M, Fig L, Zasadny K, et al. Imaging, dosimetry, and radioimmunotherapy with iodine-131-labeled anti-CD37 antibody in B-cell lymphoma. J Clin Oncol 10: 1696, 1992.

140. Kaminski MS, Gribbin T, Estes J, et al. I-131 antibody for previously untreatd follicular lymphoma: clinical and molecular remissions. Proc Am Soc Clin Oncol 17: 2a, 1998.

141. Cagnoni PJ, Ceriani RL, Cole W, et al. Phase I study of high-dose radioimmunotherapy with 90-Y-hu-BrE-3 followed by autologous stem cell support (ASCS) in patients with metastatic breast cancer. Seventh Conference on Radioimmunodetection and Radioimmunotherapy of Cancer, Princeton, NJ, 1998.

142. Slamon DJ, Clark G, Wong S, et al. Human breast cancer: correlation of relapse and survival with amplification of the Her-2/neu oncogene. Science 2235: 177-181, 1987.

143. Baselga J, Tripathy D, Mendelsohn J, et al. Phase II study of weekly intravenous recombinant humanized anti-p185^{HER2} monoclonal antibody in patients with ^{HER2}/neu-overexpressing metastatic breast cancer. J Clin Oncol 14: 737-744, 1996.

144. Slamon DL. Alteration of the HER-2/neu gene in human breast cancer: Diagnostic and therapeutic implications. Rosenthal Award Lecture at the 90th Annual Meeting of the American Association for Cancer Research (AACR), Philadelphia, PA, 1999.

145. Pegram MD, Lipton A, Hayes DF. Phase II study of receptor-enhanced chemosensitivity using recombinant humanized anti-p185$^{HER2/neu}$ monoclonal antibody plus cisplatin in patients with HER2/neu-overexpressing metastatic breast cancer refractory to chemotherapy treatment. J Clin Oncol 16: 2659-2671, 1998.

146. Slamon D, Leyland-Jones B, Shak S, et al. Addition of Herceptin9 (humanized anti-her2 antibody) to first line chemotherapy for her2 overexpressing metastatic breast cancer markedly increases anticancer activity: A randomized, multinational controlled phase III trial. Proc Am Soc Clin Oncol 17: 98a, 1998.

6

High Dose Therapy with Stem Cell Support for Breast Cancer: The Jury Is Still Out

Michael Crump, M.D.
Associate Professor of Medicine
Toronto-Sunnybrook Regional Cancer Center

Kathleen Pritchard, M.D.
Professor of Medicine
Toronto-Sunnybrook Regional Cancer Center

INTRODUCTION

The treatment of breast cancer, both in the adjuvant and metastatic setting, has been a story of great success coupled with frustration. For primary breast cancer, a series of randomized controlled trials testing new concepts in the application of chemotherapy and hormonal therapy, in both node positive and node negative patients, has produced small but significant improvements in disease-free and overall survival.[1-3] Individual trials reported recently have also indicated incremental benefit from the substitution of epirubicin for methotrexate[4,5] and the addition of paclitaxel after doxorubicin, plus cyclophosphamide (AC) chemotherapy.[6] Nonetheless, subgroups of patients, particularly those with large numbers of positive lymph nodes, appear to derive relatively limited benefit from currently available treatment and in these patients the diagnosis of breast cancer carries a high mortality.

For patients with metastatic breast cancer, currently available treatment remains palliative. It has been difficult to discern the exact magnitude of the impact of systemic therapy on survival in women with distant metastases, but current evidence suggests that the degree of survival prolongation is probably no more than six months.[7] A recent systematic overview of more than 189 randomized trials of therapy for metastatic breast cancer concluded that some, but not all, of the concepts tested resulted in prolongation of survival.[8] However, the benefits were rather modest and formal evaluation of quality of life for the large majority of these trials was not carried out. Particularly in the metastatic setting, the improvement in the outcome of patients with breast cancer has been incremental; patients and physicians alike still await the development of a "home run."

It is nearly 20 years since it was recognized that chemotherapy dose is a "critical factor"[9] in the application of systemic chemotherapy in cancer treatment. Retrospective analyses of patients receiving chemotherapy for primary and metastatic breast cancer have indicated that the delivery of chemotherapy (chemotherapy dose intensity[10] or, more recently, dose density[11]) may have a significant impact on both response rate and survival. Since the mid-1980's, a number of randomized controlled trials have been initiated to test this hypothesis, some of which are discussed below.

The experimental evidence for the existence of such a dose response relationship is substantial. Early work by Skipper and Schabel[12,13] demonstrated that higher doses of certain chemotherapeutic agents, up to a particular level, yield higher response rates in tumors. A number of high-dose chemotherapy regimens were designed based on these concepts, as well as on the demonstration of non-cross resistance between alkylating agents, and the possibility of therapeutic synergy, examined in phase I testing, and applied to patients in phase II trials. The biological basis for high-dose therapy has been discussed extensively in the literature and is reviewed elsewhere.[14,15]

A great deal of progress has been made in the understanding and application of high-dose chemotherapy with hematopoietic stem cell support, both in breast cancer as well as in a number of hematopoietic neoplasms. This treatment has been demonstrated to produce superior outcomes in patients with relapsed non-Hodgkin's lymphoma (NHL),[16] but not consistently in all reports when studied in high-risk NHL patients at the time of initial diagnosis[17,18] or acute myeloid leukemia.[19,20] The results of this treatment in other chemotherapy-sensitive diseases such as Hodgkin's disease[21,22] or testicular cancer,[23,24] are encouraging, and long-term follow-up of studies is ongoing to determine the exact impact on survival. Nevertheless, substantial technological advances in the mobilization and enumeration of hematopoietic stem cells, as well as advances in other supportive care aspects, have improved the safety of this treatment.[25-27] Because of this, high-dose therapy is now widely available for patients with breast cancer, and breast cancer is now the most common indication for peripheral blood stem cell transplant (PBSCT) reported to the North American Autologous Blood and Marrow Registry (NAABMTR).[28] An increasing proportion of patients reported to the NAABMTR are receiving this treatment in the setting of high-risk primary breast cancer, and its use in the adjuvant setting accounts for more than 50% of breast cancer transplants. Although an increasing number of patients have been receiving this treatment, few have been treated in research studies designed to test the hypothesis that high-dose therapy with stem cell support produces superior outcomes (response rate, time to progression, overall survival and quality of life) compared to standard dose approaches. A number of large randomized trials have now been completed, or are ongoing, but mature results from a number of these studies are not yet available. Should such therapy be offered as a standard treatment option for women with high-risk, node positive breast cancer, or metastatic breast cancer? We will review the current data on the application of high-dose therapy with stem cell support in the treatment of breast cancer and put forward the argument that it is still premature to draw this conclusion. The current weight of evidence does not support the argument that high-dose therapy is the "only hope" for patients with metastatic or high-risk breast cancer.

CHEMOTHERAPY DOSE INTENSITY AND OUTCOME IN BREAST CANCER

The impact of chemotherapy dose intensity (the amount of chemotherapy received compared to a reference "standard regimen" in mg/m^2 per week) was initially described by Hryniuk and Bush in 1984.[10] Similar analyses were also reported for patients treated in the adjuvant setting.[29] Because of the retrospective nature of these analyses, and because increasing chemotherapy dose increases the degree of hematologic and non-hematologic toxicity, appropriately designed randomized controlled trials have been carried out in the adjuvant and metastatic setting to formally test this hypothesis. The CALGB study reported by Wood et al.,[30] demonstrated that delivery of adequate doses of one particular anthracycline-based regimen in adjuvant treatment of node-positive breast cancer was necessary in order to achieve the best result. A similar trial by Tannock et al.[31] using CMF in metastatic breast cancer, which came to the same conclusion. However, other studies that have attempted to increase doses within conventional-dose ranges have not conclusively shown that increasing dose intensity results in improved survival or quality of life.[32-34]

It should not be concluded from these results that high-dose therapy supported by stem cells—especially the single myeloablative treatments most commonly used—would be of no value. The two strategies are sufficiently different in terms of tumor cell kinetics and cell killing, as well as pharmacokinetics and pharmacodynamics, that such comparisons are probably not justified.

RANDOMIZED TRIALS TESTING HIGH-DOSE CHEMOTHERAPY WITH STEM CELL SUPPORT IN BREAST CANCER: CURRENT RESULTS

Metastatic Breast Cancer

Stadtmauer, et al.[35] have presented data on 184 women randomized to receive high-dose chemotherapy followed by stem cell support, or maintenance chemotherapy for two years, in the Philadelphia Intergroup Study (PBT1). Patients in this study had breast cancer that was either locally recurrent or distant metastatic disease, were age less than 60 years and had no prior chemotherapy for metastatic disease. Women were required to be more than six months following completion of prior adjuvant chemotherapy, and to have received at least one prior hormonal treatment, if the original tumor was ER positive. Patients who had received < 400 mg/m^2 of adjuvant doxorubicin, received CAF for 4-6 cycles prior to response evaluation. Those who had prior doxorubicin of more than 400 mg/m^2 received CMF, with or without Prednisone for 4-6 cycles before restaging. Patients who achieved a complete or partial remission were randomized to receive high-dose cyclophosphamide, thiotepa, and carboplatin.[36] Because early in this trial bone marrow harvesting was required, bone marrow involvement with tumor was an exclusion criterion. Subsequently, the protocol was amended to allow peripheral blood stem cell collection. The ECOG Data Monitoring Committee unblinded the study in October 1998 at the second interim analysis, after 93 deaths had been observed. As of the end of March 1999, 114 deaths had been observed.

A total of 553 women were enrolled and 513 were eligible. Two hundred and ninety-six (57%) had a complete response (CR) (11% CR, 47% partial response (PR)). Approximately 90% received CAF as induction chemotherapy. One hundred and ninety-nine of the 296 responding patients were ultimately randomized (83% of CRs, 59% of PRs). Slightly more of the non-randomized responding patients had visceral disease compared to those who were randomized, whereas more of the randomized patients had had a CR to induction chemotherapy. Fifteen of the 199 randomized patients were found to be ineligible. The patient characteristics of the 184 eligible patients were well-balanced with respect to age, estrogen receptor past status, site of dominant disease and prior adjuvant chemotherapy. A somewhat greater proportion of patients assigned to transplant had a CR to induction chemotherapy (29/101, 29%), compared to 16/83 patients in the CMF maintenance arm (19%). At the time of analysis, the median follow-up of the entire group of randomized patients was 37 months. The median survival of the patients randomized to autologous stem cell transplantation (ABMT) was 24 months, compared to 26 months for the CMF arm. The three-year survival was 32% in the ABMT arm and 38% in the CMF arm (p = 0.23). Median survival for patients with a CR was the same in both arms (32 mos for ABMT, 33 mos for CMF) as was three year overall survival (42% for ABMT, 49% for CMF; p = 0.39). For patients with a PR, the corresponding median survivals were 23 and 22 mos, and three-year survival was 27 and 36% for the ABMT and CMF groups, respectively.

There was only one treatment related death of the 184 randomized patients, occurring in the ABMT arm from hepatic veno-occlusive disease. Although this is the largest randomized trial of high-dose therapy with stem cell support in chemotherapy-sensitive metastatic breast cancer reported to date, it shows no improvement in overall survival, time to progression or progression-free survival. It seems unlikely that these results will change with further follow-up. The high-dose therapy regimen used is one with which American physicians are very familiar, and was used almost in one-third of the patients reported to the NAAMBTR.[36] The treatment-related mortality, given that this was a multi-centre trial, was impressively low, and the lack of difference between the two arms cannot be attributed to toxicity of the high-dose regimen. Details regarding additional therapy following protocol therapy (such as the use of taxanes, "crossover" to delayed stem cell transplantation), were not given in this presentation. One can only speculate as to the impact of these maneuvers on the ultimate results of the trial. It would appear from this study that high-dose therapy with stem cell support, as commonly practiced in North America, does not offer any advantages to women with metastatic breast cancer.

There are considerable differences between this study and the smaller randomized study published by Bezwoda, et al.[37] In that study, patients with metastatic breast cancer who were randomized to the high-dose arm were treated with high-dose chemotherapy for two cycles as initial treatment. In addition, high-dose cyclophosphamide, 60 mg/kg, was used for stem cell mobilization on both occasions, amounting, more or less, to four cycles of high-dose alkylating agent therapy. Progression free survival and overall survival in that study were superior in the high-dose arm compared to that in women receiving six doses of cyclophosphamide, mitoxantrone and 5-FU.

There have been numerous criticisms of the Bezwoda trial. In that study women with estrogen receptor positive tumors who had responded to chemotherapy were placed on tamoxifen. Because the overall and complete response rate was higher in the high-dose therapy arm, more patients in that arm were assigned to tamoxifen, possibly favorably influencing time to progression and disease-free survival. It is even possible that this bias in tamoxifen assignment could ultimately affect survival given the non-random nature of the tamoxifen assignment. The time to progression and survival on the standard dose arm was very short. This chemotherapy regimen has been criticized, but a number of randomized trials comparing doxorubicin versus mitoxantrone in combination with cyclophosphamide and 5-FU have shown no difference in response rates or overall survival.[33] A recent exception to this, by Stewart et al.,[38] showed a significant difference in both response rate, time to progression and overall survival favoring the doxorubicin-containing arm. Whether or not the control group in the Bezwoda trial would have faired better with doxorubicin containing chemotherapy, or the inclusion of a taxane at progression, is unknown. This study does support a number of the principles of high-dose chemotherapy, but leaves many questions unanswered.

Lotz et al. reported the result of the French protocol PEGASE 04.[39] This study enrolled a small number of women, 61, with metastatic breast cancer from September 1992 and December 1996. One-third had de-novo metastatic breast cancer and the rest were treated at first relapse. In this trial, women were randomized after 4-6 cycles of conventional dose chemotherapy to receive high dose mitoxantrone 45 mg/m^2, cyclophosphamide 120 mg/kg and melphalan 140 mg/m^2, or to continue the same chemotherapy. Progression-free survival at two years is superior in the high dose arm compared to standard dose therapy (26.9 vs 15.6 months, p =0.04), but there is no difference in median overall survival (36.1 vs 15.7 months, p =0.08). The power to detect a meaningful prolongation of survival in this study is obviously limited and further follow-up would be of interest.

Investigators from Duke University have reported the results of a randomized trial of high-dose cyclophosphamide, cisplatin and BCNU followed by ABMT compared to no further therapy, in previously untreated women with metastatic breast cancer.[40] All women in this trial received induction therapy with doxorubicin, methotrexate and 5-FU, a regimen that has previously been reported by these investigators to produce a high CR rate. Only patients with a CR were randomized and patients with bony disease were excluded. Most of the women who were randomized had soft tissue disease. Disease-free survival was significantly higher for patients randomized to immediate consolidation with ABMT (median 1.8 vs 0.3 yrs; p = 0.002), however, patients randomized to initial observation followed by ABMT at relapse had a better overall survival than those transplanted immediately (3.2 vs 1.7 yrs; p = 0.04). These data are somewhat surprising at first glance and difficult to reconcile with the pre-clinical data and previous experience with ABMT after failure of chemotherapy for metastatic breast cancer. One explanation that has been offered is that delay in the administration of high-dose therapy permits reversal of multi-drug resistance in the residual tumor cell population, therefore making them more susceptible to later treatment with high-dose chemotherapy. Although there may be theoretical support for this argument, prolonged survival has not been the experience when patients who have had multiple chemotherapy regiments for breast cancer undergo ABMT, and it contradicts data from a number of more chemotherapy-sensitive diseases where ABMT has prolonged survival.

These observations pose considerable challenges in designing further randomized trials to test the role of induction chemotherapy, as well as the exact timing of high-dose treatment in the management of metastatic breast cancer. In addition, data recently reported from the NAABMTR shed light on prognostic factors that may have a significant influence on outcome after ABMT for metastatic breast cancer.[41] In this retrospective analysis of 1188 women reported from 63 centres in the United States and Canada, factors associated with a significant risk of treatment failure were age >45 years, performance status <90%, absence of hormone receptors, prior use of adjuvant chemotherapy, initial disease-free survival after adjuvant therapy <18 months, liver or CNS metastases, 3 or more sites of metastatic disease and incomplete response to induction chemotherapy. Women with no risk factors had a three-year probability of remaining progression-free of 43%, compared to 4% for women with 3 or more risk factors. Prognostic factors predicting outcome after doxorubicin, 5-FU and methotrexate induction therapy (AFM) followed by ABMT were very similar in a recent report from Duke University.[41a] These prognostic factors are strikingly similar to those for metastatic breast cancer treated with conventional dose therapy but nonetheless should be taken into account in the design of future trials and in the interpretation.

In 1996, the National Cancer Institute of Canada Clinical Trials Group (NCIC-CTG) embarked on a randomized trial of high-dose therapy with stem cell support in patients with responding metastatic breast cancer. This trial was undertaken because of the uncertainty created by the Bezwoda and Peters studies. In addition, it was clear that the standard of care for metastatic breast cancer was heterogeneous and the addition of many new drugs to the oncologist armamentarium was having an influence on palliative endpoints such as response and potentially also on quality of life. It was therefore felt that the appropriate control arm for such a comparative study should reflect the patient's treatment history and regional differences in the application of cytotoxic agents in metastatic breast cancer. In this way the control arm is an accurate reflection of the currently available systemic therapy options for the treatment of metastatic breast cancer.

In the NCIC-CTG MA.16 study, women with locoregional recurrence or distant metastases, who are responding to their first chemotherapy for metastatic breast cancer, are randomized after four cycles to an additional two cycles of induction treatment followed by stem cell collection; or to continuing the same chemotherapy used during induction, depending on the induction regimen used. Women in the standard dose arm are treated to a total dose of 450 mg/m^2 of doxorubicin or 840 mg/m^2 of epirubicin. Patients receiving a taxane as induction chemotherapy who are assigned to the standard therapy arm will receive a total of at least 8 or 9 cycles of treatment. Women in the high-dose arm receive high-dose cyclophosphamide, mitoxantrone and carboplatin followed by stem cell infusion. Those with breast cancer which is ER positive who have not previously progressed on tamoxifen, are given this drug upon completion of chemotherapy; those who had been previously exposed to tamoxifen may be given an aromatase inhibitor at their physician's discretion. The use of local radiation treatment for solitary soft tissue or bony sites is encouraged in both arms, but mandated in the stem cell transplant arm. The use of bisphosphonates for patients with bone metastases is encouraged in both arms.

The primary endpoint of the NCIC-CTG trial is overall survival. Other endpoints being evaluated are time to progression and, importantly, quality of life comparison between the two arms. This study has the power to detect a 15% difference in overall survival at two years and requires a total of 192 patients to be randomized. This accrual target was met in July 1999, just over two years after the study opened. Sufficient events for analysis of survival are expected by mid-2000.

**High Dose Therapy as Part of
Adjuvant Therapy for High-Risk Primary Breast Cancer**

It is still widely regarded that tumor size and nodal status are the most important prognostic factors in the treatment of breast cancer. Several groups have reported poor long-term outcome in patients with high numbers of positive lymph nodes at the time of surgery. In an effort to improve on these results, investigators in the 1980's performed investigations of high-dose therapy with stem cell support in this patient population. Compared to historical controls, women receiving high-dose therapy with stem cell support appear to have improved disease-free and overall survival. Updated data from Peters et al.[42] have indicated that approximately two-thirds of women with 10 or more positive lymph nodes who receive conventional dose CAF chemotherapy, followed by high-dose cyclophosphamide, cisplatin and BCNU supported by bone marrow and PBSCs, are alive and disease-free more than six years from transplant. Using a somewhat different approach, Gianni et al.[43] have shown that high-dose sequential treatment provides superior results compared to conventional-dose treatment with sequential doxorubicin followed by CMF using non-randomized controls. In this strategy, investigators from the Milan Cancer Institute showed that maximally tolerated doses of individual agents, supported by hematopoietic growth factors or autologous stem cells, appeared to result in an improved outcome, a strategy which they have shown is superior in a randomized study in patients with NHL.[44] The results from these two phase II breast cancer trials led to the widespread adoption of high-dose therapy with stem cell support for women with high risk, node positive breast cancer, despite the lack of data from randomized trials.

As impressive as these early results were, it became clear that one reason for the observed improvement in outcome was the nature of patient selection and the influence of stage migration. Patients who enter into studies of high-dose therapy are frequently required to have extensive staging with CT scans of head, chest, abdomen and pelvis as well as bone marrow biopsies, to ensure that such patients do not already have metastatic breast cancer. This degree of evaluation is considerably more than was required in the clinical trials from which the historical control populations are derived.

We initially reported that 23% of patients referred for participation in a randomized trial of high-dose therapy with stem cell support (CALGB 9082; NCIC CTG MA 13), who had normal chest X-ray, bone scan and ultrasound, were subsequently found to have metastatic disease after more rigorous investigation.[45] We have expanded this evaluation to include 133 women referred for possible inclusion in that randomized trial. Twenty-four women declined to participate in the study and were not screened further. Ten were found to have metastatic breast cancer at the time of referral, based on clinical examination or review of original radiology, and these women were not evaluated further. A total of 88 women completed all required staging evaluations (CT scans of the head, chest, abdomen and pelvis and bilateral bone marrow biopsies). Metastatic breast cancer was discovered after more extensive staging in 15 of these women (17%; 95%; CI 10-24%). Sites of metastases were bone marrow (n = 5), pulmonary parenchyma (n = 4), internal mammary nodes (n = 3), liver (n = 2) and bone (n = 1). Since such patients would have been expected to ultimately progress after adjuvant chemotherapy, their exclusion from a cohort of high-risk patients would in turn increase the disease-free survival and possibly overall survival of such a patient cohort. The actual extent to which this "stage migration" contributes to an improvement in overall outcome is unclear.

Other authors have also reported selection bias in phase II studies of ABMT for breast cancer. Garcia-Carbonera et al.[46] performed a retrospective analysis of patients with 10 or more positive lymph nodes treated with conventional chemotherapy, and found that those who met standard selection criteria for high-dose therapy (age < 60 years, no significant co-morbid disease and no progression during adjuvant treatment) had a significantly better outcome than those who did not meet these criteria. In a multivariate analysis that included age, menopausal status, tumor size, number of involved lymph nodes, grade, HDCT criteria and the use of locoregional radiation treatment, only the latter two variables had a significant impact on disease-free or overall survival. Rahman et al.[47] reported a similar analysis, in women with metastatic breast cancer, indicating a superior outcome for patients who would have met conventional criteria for high-dose therapy compared to those who would not. Taken together, it appears that patients enrolled in high-dose therapy studies may have an intrinsically superior prognosis, for one reason or another, compared to historical controls receiving conventional dose treatment. These analyses underlie the hazard of relying on historical controls when comparing the results of high-dose therapy to those of conventional dose treatment.

A number of randomized trials of high-dose therapy in the adjuvant setting are underway or have been completed. Early results from some of those studies are now available. Two of these trials are small, randomizing approximately 80 patients each, and are significantly underpowered to detect anything but a very large difference between standard therapy and high-dose treatment. The study from the Netherlands Cancer Institute[48] in particular has other design features that make generalization difficult. Patients in that study were required to have a positive infraclavicular lymph node biopsy (level III lymph node involvement) before proceeding with preoperative chemotherapy, surgery and randomization to either one additional cycle of conventional dose treatment, or high-dose cyclophosphamide, thiotepa and carboplatin. These investigators pointed out that all patients in their study, regardless of the arm to which they were randomized, appear to be doing better than previous historical controls receiving the same chemotherapy and locoregional treatment. The relevance of these data to the clinical setting described in most phase II reports, where patients have undergone conventional breast cancer surgery with axillary dissection, remains to be seen.

At the most recent meeting of the American Society of Clinical Oncology, preliminary results from three other randomized trials were presented. Professor Bezwoda from South Africa reported a study of a similar design to his previously described trial in metastatic breast cancer.[49] Patients at high risk of recurrence in the current study included those with 10 or more lymph nodes involved; women with T3a, ER negative tumors with seven or more positive nodes; or any tumor size with seven or more nodes involved, if the patient had two first degree relatives with breast cancer. All women were less than 55 years of age, and were staged with a chest X-ray, abdominal ultrasound and bone scan. Standard chemotherapy consisted of CAF or CEF given intravenously every three weeks for six cycles. The high dose chemotherapy was similar to that reported by this group previously: two cycles of cyclophosphamide 4.4 g/m^2, mitoxantrone 45 mg/m^2 and etoposide 1.5 g/m^2, with an interval of 28-42 days between courses. In this trial, stem cells were collected using G-CSF alone and were not cryopreserved. Stem cells for the second high-dose treatment were mobilized with G-CSF following recovery from the first high-dose treatment. With a median follow-up of 5.3 years, overall survival for the 75 patients in the high-dose arm is significantly better than that for the 79 women in the standard dose arm (p < 0.05), as is relapse free survival (p < 0.05). A similar degree of cardiac toxicity was noted, and there was one death from treatment before 150 days in both arms of this study. Although this trial is small, freedom from relapse and mortality are significantly improved in the high-dose arm. **[Editor's Note: The Bezwoda study has come under scrutiny because of allegations of scientific misconduct.]** These results should make investigators re-consider the value of conventional dose "induction chemotherapy " as well as to the wisdom of using a single cycle of high-dose chemotherapy treatment in a solid tumor such as breast cancer.

There were two other studies reported, on the other hand, which did not show improvement in survival. One of these was from the Scandinavian Breast Cancer Study Group comparing high-dose cyclophosphamide, thiotepa and carboplatin with stem cell support to repeated doses of escalated 5-FU, epirubicin and cyclophosphamide.[50] This study included women under the age of 60, with eight or more positive lymph nodes, or those with five or more positive lymph nodes whose tumor was estrogen receptor negative and/or had a high S-phase fraction. Patients enrolled in this study were somewhat different from the usual adjuvant population, however. Also eligible were patients with positive bone scans (where the accompanying bone x-rays were negative for metastases); those with abnormal liver function tests and those with micrometastases found on bone marrow biopsy. These investigators had previously reported a lack of relationship between pharmacokinetic parameters for the individual drugs in the CEF regimen and body surface area; therefore, dosing of CEF in the "standard arm" was based on the nadir neutrophil and platelet counts during the previous cycle. Escalated doses of CEF were supported by G-CSF and a total of nine cycles were given. All patients in both arms received locoregional radiotherapy and tamoxifen 20 mg a day for five years. At the time of reporting, in April 1999, the median follow-up of the 525 women enrolled in this study was four years. At the time of reporting, there had been more relapses in the autologous transplant arm (92) compared to the escalated FEC arm (66). Overall, there was more grade 3 or 4 toxicity reported in the ABMT arm, but of concern was the development of eight cases of secondary myeloid malignancies (3 MDS, 5 AML) in the FEC arm, an incidence of 3.9%. The "standard" arm in this trial sought to maximize dose intensity, and delivered more chemotherapy than the "single dose" arm. The lack of a control arm makes the result somewhat difficult to interpret, as does the inclusion of patients with low volume metastatic disease. In addition, the duration of follow-up in this study is quite short, and additional information about quality of life and long-term toxicity is awaited.

The third study presented was a preliminary report of a prospective randomized comparison of two doses of combination alkylating agents as consolidation after CAF chemotherapy in high risk primary breast cancer.[51] Eligible patients had stage II or IIIa breast cancer involving 10 or more positive nodes, clear surgical margins and were required to have normal CT scans of the head, chest, abdomen and pelvis, and negative bilateral bone marrow biopsies by light microscopy. After four cycles of cyclophosphamide, doxorubicin and 5-FU patients were randomized to receive high-dose cyclophosphamide 5625 mg/m^2, cisplatin 165 mg/m^2 and BCNU 600 mg/m^2 (CPB) with bone marrow and peripheral blood stem cell support; or intermediate dose CPB consisting of cyclophosphamide 900 mg/m^2, cisplatin 90 mg/m^2 and BCNU 90 mg/m^2 with G-CSF support if needed. All patients were planned for locoregional radiotherapy, and patients with hormone receptor positive cancer received tamoxifen for five years. A total of 874 women were enrolled and 783 randomized; 91 who were not randomized included 22 who developed recurrent breast cancer while on therapy, two who died due to CAF toxicity, 26 patients who did not have insurance coverage for ABMT, 20 who withdrew and 21 who were found to be ineligible. The median follow-up at the time of reporting is 37 months. Using an intent to treat analysis, there was no difference in event-free survival between high dose and intermediate dose CPB (68% vs 64%); similarly there was no difference in overall survival (78% vs 80%). Fewer patients in the high-dose therapy arm who have relapsed compared to the intermediate dose arm (21.6% vs 32.2%), however, high-dose therapy was associated with 29 treatment-related deaths compared to none in the intermediate dose arm. At this point in time, there is no difference in overall survival between the two arms. Further follow-up of this trial is necessary and the data are not considered to be mature. It is clear from this study that mortality from high-dose therapy is not isolated to the first 100 days after transplant (it was 3% at 100 days but 7% at one year), and that these events have had a significant bearing on the outcome of the high-dose therapy group. Additional follow-up is clearly needed to see whether the trend towards reduction in disease recurrence in the high dose arm is maintained and to evaluate the long-term impact of this therapy on survival.

**High-Dose Chemotherapy with
Stem Cell Support: The Jury Is Still Out**

A number of significant questions remain as to the place of high dose therapy in women with breast cancer. Mature data from randomized trials of induction therapy followed by myeloablative doses of chemotherapy do not support the tenant that "more is better," except when used up-front without induction therapy. Even in the optimum group of patients—those who have had a complete response to induction treatment—there was no difference noted in disease-free or overall survival between high-dose therapy and maintenance CMF seen in the Intergroup study reported by Stadtmauer et al.[35] A large, methodologically sound confirmatory randomized trial testing the up-front approach reported by Bezwoda et al.[37] is urgently needed. As part of adjuvant therapy for women judged to be at high risk of disease recurrence, the randomized trials to date evaluating the role of ABMT have either been too small to identify a difference,[48,52] have delivered more therapy in the "standard" arm,[50] or do not have sufficient follow-up.[51] The patient populations studied, screening evaluation prior to enrollment, and treatments received also are quite heterogeneous (Table 1), making comparisons between the trials difficult. One must conclude that this therapy remains to be proven in this setting and should not be offered to women outside of *comparative* trials. Additional data from the Intergroup trial reported by Peters et al and from the ECOG-SWOG comparison of six cycles of CAF to six cycles of CAF followed by high-dose cyclophosphamide and thiotepa (ECOG 2190) are required before the impact of this treatment on survival—and the long-term effects accompanying it—can be properly assessed.

On the other hand, the data reported by Bezwoda are intriguing and suggest directions for future trial design. Although the small phase II trials of multiple cycles of high-dose therapy following standard dose induction treatment have not convincingly shown a benefit to the addition of a second cycle of ablative treatment, the randomized trials reported from South Africa have been consistent in showing a survival advantage to this treatment when used up-front without induction.[37,49] **[Editor's Note: The Bezwoda study has come under scrutiny because of allegations of scientific misconduct.]** If dose intensity is truly an important concept in the systemic treatment of breast cancer, other than determining the optimum dose of a particular regimen to be given in the outpatient setting,[30] then a better test would be to use the concepts demonstrated by these prospective trials and the retrospective comparison by

Gianni et al.[43]   At least one such randomized trial has completed accrual, performed by the International Breast Cancer Study Group (IBCSG 15-95). Pilot data, upon which this trial was based, showed that it is safe and feasible to administer three cycles of very high-dose cyclophosphamide and epirubicin (CE) supported by an infusion of peripheral blood stem cells and G-CSF for three cycles every 21 days.[53]   The long-term results of this approach in unscreened women with high-risk breast cancer appear to be at least equivalent to those achieved with induction therapy followed by ABMT. If the randomized study comparing multiple cycles of high dose CE is positive, it would confirm the South African data and reshape the way we think of dose-intensity. It is important that comparative trials incorporating this strategy for delivering "dose-intensive" chemotherapy should be undertaken in the metastatic setting as well.

        Treatment of breast cancer continues to evolve, and high-dose therapy must be considered a treatment in evolution. Small gains in survival have been achieved by the addition of new agents such as paclitaxel, herceptin, taxotere and even, potentially, aromatase inhibitors and bisphosphonates in either the adjuvant or metastatic settings. In addition to the data that has emerged from studies of high-dose therapy to date, the information about the role of these new agents in improving outcome must be incorporated into future study designs of high-dose therapy, in order for patients and physicians to understand the place of the latter in the management of breast cancer.

REFERENCES

1.   Early Breast Cancer Trialists Collaborative Group: Polychemotherapy for early breast cancer: An overview of the randomized trials. Lancet 352: 930-942,1998.
2.   Early Breast Cancer Trialists Collaborative Group: Tamoxifen for early breast cancer: An overview of the randomized trials. Lancet 351: 1451-1467,1998.
3.   Early Breast Cancer Trialists Collaborative Group: Ovarian ablation for early breast cancer: An overview of the randomized trials. Lancet 348:1189-1196, 1996.
4.   Levine MN, Bramwell VH, Pritchard KI, Norris BD, Shepherd LE, et al: Randomized trial of intensive cyclophosphamide, epirubicin, and fluorouracil in premenopausal women with node-positive breast cancer.

National Cancer Institute of Canada Clinical Trials Group. J Clin Oncol 16(8): 2651-2658, 1998.

5. Mouridsen HT, Andersen J, Andersson M, Dombernowsky P, et al: Adjuvant anthracycline in breast cancer. Improved outcome in premenopausal patients following substitution of methotrexate in the CMF combination with epirubicin. Proc Am Soc Clin Oncol 18: 68a, 1999. (abst # 254).

6. Henderson IC, Berry D, Demetri G, et al: Improved disease-free and overall survival from the addition of sequential paclitaxel but not from the escalation of doxorubicin dose level in the adjuvant chemotherapy of patients with node-positive primary breast cancer. Proc Am Soc Clin Oncol 17:101a, 1998. (abst # 390A).

7. Henderson IC, Garber JE, Breitmeyer JB, Hayes DF, Harris JR: Comprehensive management of disseminated breast cancer. Cancer 66:1439-1448, 1990.

8. Fossati R, Confalonieri C, Torri V, Ghyislandi TE, Penna A, Pistotti V, Tinazzi A, Liberati A: Cytotoxic and hormonal treatment for metastatic breast cancer: A systematic review of published randomized trials involving 31,510 women. J Clin Oncol 16:3439-3460, 1998.

9. Frei, III E, Canellos GP: Dose: A critical factor in cancer chemotherapy. Am J Med 69:585-594, 1980.

10. Hryniuk W, Bush H: The importance of dose intensity in cancer chemotherapy of metastatic breast cancer. J Clin Oncol 2:1281-1288, 1984.

11. Hudis C, Seidman A, Beselga J, et al: Sequential dose-dense doxorubicin, paclitaxel and cyclophosphamide for resectable high-risk breast cancer: Feasibility and efficacy. J Clin Oncol 17:93-100, 1999.

12. Skipper HE: Laboratory models: The historical perspective. Cancer Treat Rep 70:3-7, 1986.

13. Skipper HE, Schabel FM, Jary R, Wilcox WS. Experimental evaluation of antitumor agents. Cancer Chemother Rep 35:1-34,1964.

14. Frei, III E, Antman K, Teicher B, Eder P, Schnipper L: Bone marrow autotransplantation for solid tumors – prospects. J Clin Oncol 7:515-526, 1989.

15. Henderson IC, Hayes DF, Gelman R: Dose-response in the treatment of breast cancer: A critical review. J Clin Oncol 6:1501-1515, 1988.

16. Philip T, Guglielmi C, Hagenbeek A, et al: Autologous bone marrow transplantation as compared with standard chemotherapy in relapses of

chemotherapy sensitive non-Hodgkin's lymphoma. N Engl J Med 332:1045-1051, 1995.

17. Haioun C, Lepage E, Gisselbrecht C, et al: Comparison of autologous bone marrow transplantation with sequential chemotherapy for intermediate-grade and high-grade non-Hodgkin's lymphoma in first complete remission: A study of 464 patients. J Clin Oncol 12:2543-2551, 1994.

18. Verdonck LF, Van Putten WLJ, Hagenbeek A, et al: Comparison of CHOP chemotherapy with autologous bone marrow transplantation for slowly responding patients with aggressive non-Hodgkin's lymphoma. N Engl J Med 333:1540-1051, 1995.

19. Burnett AK, Goldstone AH, Stevens RMF, et al: Randomized comparison of addition of autologous bone marrow transplantation to intensive chemotherapy for acute myeloid leukemia in first remission: Results of MRC AML 10 trial. Lancet 351:700-709, 1998.

20. Cassileth RA, Harrington DP, Appelbaum FP, et al: Chemotherapy compared with autologous or allogeneic bone marrow transplantation in the management of acute myeloid leukemia in first remission. New Engl J Med 339:1649-1656, 1998.

21. Linch DC, Winfield D, Goldstone AH, Moir D, Hancock B, McMillan A, Chopra R, Milligan D, Hudson GV: Dose intensification with autologous bone-marrow transplantation in relapsed and resistant Hodgkin's disease: results of a BNLI randomized trial. Lancet 341:1051-1054, 1993.

22. Schmitz N, Sextro M, Pfistner D, Hasenclever H, et al: High-dose therapy (HDT) followed by hematopoietic stem cell transplantation (HSCT) for relapsed chemosensitive Hodgkin's disease (HD): Final results of a randomized GHSG and EBMT Trial (HD-R1). . Proc Am Assoc Clin Oncol 18:2a, 1999 (Abst #5).

23. Beyer J, Kingreen D, Krause M, Schleicher, et al: Long term survival of patients with recurrent or refractory germ cell tumors after high dose chemotherapy. Cancer 79: 161-168, 1997.

24. Motzer RJ, Mazumdar M, Bosl GJ, Bajorin D, et al: High-dose carboplatin, etoposide, and cyclophosphamide for patients with refractory germ cell tumors: treatment results and prognostic factors for survival and toxicity. J Clin Oncol 14: 1098-1105, 1996.

25. Schmidt N, Lynch DC, Dreger P et al. Randomized trial of filgrastim-mobilized peripheral blood progenitor cell transplantation versus autologous bone marrow transplantation in lymphoma patients. Lancet 347:353-357, 1996.

26. Dercksen MW, Rodenhuis S, Dirkson MKA, et al. Subsets of CD34+ cells and rapid hematologic recovery after peripheral blood stem cell transplantation. J Clin Oncol 13:1922-1932, 1995.

27. Shpall EJ, Wheeler CA, Turner SA, et al. A randomized phase 3 study of peripheral blood progenitor cell mobilization with stem cell factor and filgrastim in high-risk breast cancer patients. Blood 93:2491-2501, 1999.

28. Antman KH, Rowlings A, Vaughan WP, Pelz CJ, Fay JW, et al: High-dose chemotherapy with autologous hematopoietic stem-cell support for breast cancer in North America. J Clin Oncol 15:1870-1879, 1997.

29. Hryniuk W, Levine MN: Analysis of dose intensity for adjuvant chemotherapy trials in stage II breast cancer. J Clin Oncol 4:1162-1170, 1986.

30. Wood WC, Budman DR, Korzun AH, et al: Dose and dose intensity of adjuvant chemotherapy for stage II, node positive breast carcinoma. N Engl J Med 330:1253-1259, 1994.

31. Tannock IF, Boyd NF, De Boer G, et al: A randomised trial of two dose levels of cyclophosphamide, methotrexate and fluorouracil chemotherapy for patients with metastatic breast cancer. J Clin Oncol 6:1377-1387, 1988.

32. Focan C, Andrien JM, Closon MTK, et al: Dose response relationship of epirubicin based first line chemotherapy for advanced breast cancer: a prospective randomised trial. J Clin Oncol 11:1253-1263, 1993.

33. Blomqvist K, Elomma I, Rissanen P, et al: Influence of treatment schedule on toxicity and efficacy of cyclophosphamide, epirubicin, and flurouracil in metastatic breast cancer: a randomised trial comparing weekly and every 4 week administration. J Clin Oncol 11:467-473, 1993.

34. Bastholt L, Dalmark M, Gjedde SB, et al: Dose-response relationship of epirubicin in the treatment of postmenopausal women with metastatic breast cancer: a randomized study of epirubicin at four different dose levels performed by the Danish Breast Cancer Cooperative Group. J Clin Oncol 14:1146-1155, 1996.

35. Stadtmauer EA, O'Neill A, Goldstein LJ, Crilley P, et al: Phase III randomized trial of high-dose chemotherapy and stem cell support shows no difference in overall survival or severe toxicity compared to maintenance chemotherapy with cyclophosphamide, methotrexate and 5-fluorouracil for women with metastatic breast cancer who are responding to conventional induction chemotherapy: The "Philadelphia" Intergroup study. Proc Am Assoc Clin Oncol 18:1a, 1999 (Abst #1).

36.   Antman K, Ayash L, Elias A, et al: A phase II study of high-dose cyclophosphamide, thiotepa and carboplatin with autologous marrow support in women with measurable advanced breast cancer responding to standard-dose therapy. J Clin Oncol 10:102-110, 1992.

37.   Bezwoda WR, Seymour L, Dansey RD: High-dose chemotherapy with hematopoietic rescue as primary treatment for metastatic breast cancer: A randomized trial. J Clin Oncol 13:2483-2489, 1995.

38.   Stewart DJ, Evans WK, Shepherd FA, Wilson KS, Pritchard KI, Trudeau ME, Wilson JJ, Martz K: Cyclophosphamide and fluorouracil combined with mitoxantrone versus doxorubicin for breast cancer: Superiority of doxorubicin. J Clin Oncol 15:1897-1905, 1997.

39.   Lotz J-P, Cure H, Janvier M, Morvan F, et al: High-dose chemotherapy (HD-CT) with hematopoietic stem cells transplantation (HSCT) for metastatic breast cancer (MBC): Results of the French protocol PEGASE 04). Proc Am Soc Clin Oncol 18: 43a, 1999. (abst # 161).

40.   Peters WP, Jones RB, Vredenburgh JJ, et al: A large, prospective randomized trial of high-dose combination alkylating agents (CPB) with autologous cellular support (ABMS) as consolidation for patients with metastatic breast cancer achieving complete remission after intensive doxorubicin-based induction therapy (AFM). Breast Cancer Res Treat 37: 11, 1996 (abstract 11).

41.   Rowlings PA, Williams SF, Antman KH, et al.: Factors correlated with progression-free survival after high-dose chemotherapy and hematopoietic stem cell transplantation for metastatic breast cancer. JAMA 282:1335-1343, 1999.

41a. Rizzieri DA, Vredenburgh JJ, Jones R, et al.: Prognostic and predictive factors for patients with metastatic breast cancer undergoing aggressive induction therapy followed by high-dose chemotherapy with autologous stem cell support. J Clin Oncol 17:3064-3074, 1999.

42.   Peters WP, Ross M, Vredenburgh JJ, Meisenberg B, et al.: High-dose chemotherapy and autologous bone marrow support as consolidation after standard-dose adjuvant therapy for high-risk primary breast cancer. J Clin Oncol 11: 1132-1143.

42a. Peters WP, Berry D, Vredenburgh JJ, et al.: Five year follow-up of high-dose combination alkylating agents with ABMT as consolidation after standard-dose CAF for primary breast cancer involving >10 axillary lymph nodes (Duke/CALGB 8782). Proc Am Soc Clin Oncol 14:316, 1995 (Abstr 933).

43. Gianni AM, Siena M, Bregni M, et al: Efficacy, toxicity and applicability of high-dose sequential chemotherapy as adjuvant treatment in operable breast cancer with 10 or more involved axillary nodes: Five year results. J Clin Oncol 15: 1812-2321, 1997.

44. Gianni AM, Bregni M, Siena, et al: High-dose chemotherapy and autologous bone marrow transplantation compared with MACOP-B in aggressive B cell lymphoma. N Engl J Med 336: 1290-1297, 1997.

45. Crump M, Goss PE, Prince M, Girouard C: Outcome of extensive evaluation before adjuvant therapy in women with breast cancer and 10 or more positive axillary lymph nodes. J Clin Oncol 14: 66-69, 1996.

46. Garcia-Carbonera R, Hidalgo M, Paz-Ares L, Calzas J, Gomez H, Guerra JA, Hitt R, Hornedo J, Colomer R, Corets-Funes H: Patient selection in high-dose chemotherapy trials: Relevance in high-risk breast cancer. J Clin Oncol 15:3178-3184, 1997.

47. Rahman ZU, Frye DK, Buzdar AU, Smith TL, Asmar L, Champlin RE, Hortobagyi GN: Impact of selection process on response rate and long-term survival of potential high-dose chemotherapy candidates treated with standard-dose doxorubicin-containing chemotherapy in patients with metastatic breast cancer. J Clin Oncol 15:3171-3177, 1997.

48. Rodenhuis S, Richel DJ, van der Wall E, Schornagel JH, et al: Randomised trial of high-dose chemotherapy and haemopoietic progenitor-cell support in operable breast cancer with extensive axillary lymph-node involvement. Lancet 352: 515-521, 1998.

49. Bezwoda WR: Randomised controlled trial of high dose chemotherapy versus standard dose chemotherapy for high risk, surgically treated, primary breast cancer. Proc Am Assoc Clin Oncol 18:2a, 1999 (Abst #4).

50. The Scandinavian Breast Cancer Study Group 9401: Results from a randomized adjuvant breast cancer study with high dose chemotherapy with CTC, supported by autologous bone marrow stem cells versus dose escalated and tailored FEC therapy. Proc Am Assoc Clin Oncol 18:2a, 1999 (Abst #3).

51. Peters W, Rosner G, Vredenburgh J: A prospective, randomized comparison of two doses of combination alkylating agents as consolidation after CAF in high-risk primary breast cancer involving ten or more axillary lymph nodes: Preliminary results of CALGB 9082/SWOG 9114/NCIC MA.13. . Proc Am Assoc Clin Oncol 18:1a, 1999 (Abst #2).

52. Hortobagyi G, Buzdar A, Champlin R, et al.: Lack of efficacy of adjuvant high-dose (HD) tandem combination chemotherapy (CT) for high-risk

primary breast cancer (HRPBC) – A randomized trial. Proc am Soc Clin Oncol 18:471, 1998 (abstr 471).

53.   Basser RL, To LB, Collins JP, et al.: Multicycle high-dose chemotherapy and filgrastim-mobilized peripheral-blood progenitor cells in women with high-risk stage II or III breast cancer: five-year follow-up. J Clin Oncol 17:82-92, 1999.

Table 1. Characteristics of Recently Reported Randomized Trials of High-Dose Therapy in Primary Breast Cancer

Study	Patient Population	Staging	High-Dose Arm	Control Arm
Netherlands[48]	Positive level III nodes (infraclavicular node biopsy +*ve*)	Chest X-ray Ultrasound Bone scan	CTCb	FEC x 1
Scandinavian[50]	≥8 nodes +*ve* ≥5 nodes +*ve* + ER –*ve* or high S-phase	Chest X-ray Ultrasound Bone scan Bone marrow bx	CTCb	Escalated FEC x 9
South Africa[49]	T1-3a, ≥ 10+ nodes T3a, ER –*ve*, ≥7 +*ve* nodes ≥7 nodes +*ve*; +*ve* family hx	Chest X-ray Ultrasound Bone scan	CNVP x 2	FAC x 6
North American Intergroup[52]	Stage II, IIIa ≥10 nodes +*ve*	CT scans of head, chest, abd/pelvis Bilateral bone marrow bx	High-dose CPB	"standard" dose CPB

7

Preoperative Chemotherapy for Operable Breast Cancer

Eleftherios P. Mamounas, M.D.
Clinical Assistant Professor in Surgery
Case Western Reserve University

Bernard Fisher, M.D.
Distinguished Service Professor
University of Pittsburgh

INTRODUCTION

During the past 25 years, there has been a significant change in the way in which operable breast cancer is managed. As a result of laboratory and clinical investigations conducted during the 1960s, evidence was obtained that challenged Halstedian principles of tumor dissemination and provided support for an alternative hypothesis.[1] Findings from subsequent randomized clinical trials demonstrated that the extent of surgical resection had no effect on the patient's outcome[2] and that the administration of systemic therapy after surgery significantly improved the disease-free survival (DFS) and survival of such patients.[3] Consequently, there was a shift in emphasis away from surgery as the sole treatment for breast cancer, and systemic therapy became an integral part of the management of the disease.

Subsequent to the adoption of the use of systemic adjuvant therapy, a variety of circumstances occurred that eventually gave rise to the consideration that preoperative systemic therapy might result in a better patient outcome than that which resulted from the same therapy given after operation. Hypotheses formulated from findings obtained in laboratory investigations, results observed after the use of preoperative chemotherapy in the treatment of a variety of locally advanced cancers, and the advent of the use of lumpectomy for the surgical treatment of patients with operable breast cancer all provided the impetus for that thesis. Skipper et al.[4] contended that the magnitude of response of a primary tumor to chemotherapy need not reflect the response of micrometastases. Goldie and Coldman[5] suggested that, as a tumor cell population increases, an ever-expanding number of drug-resistant phenotypic variants arise due to spontaneous somatic mutations that become more difficult to eradicate. Finally, Fisher et al.[6,7] observed that primary tumor removal resulted in kinetic perturbation of micrometastases that could be abrogated by the administration of chemotherapy before tumor removal. These hypotheses were instrumental in providing a rationale for the evaluation of preoperative therapy.

Another basis for evaluating the worth of preoperative chemotherapy related to the observation that when such therapy was administered for the treatment of a variety of locally advanced tumors, including breast cancer,[8-13] it resulted in tumor shrinkage and, thus, allowed for less mutilating surgery. Not, however, until the efficacy of lumpectomy was demonstrated in patients with operable breast cancer was there increased interest in the idea of using preoperative chemotherapy to treat the disease.[14,15] When it was shown that such therapy induced shrinkage of large primary operable tumors, thus making lumpectomy possible in women who would otherwise have had a mastectomy,[16-18] further evaluation of preoperative chemotherapy became necessary. In order to justify the use of preoperative chemotherapy, it was necessary to determine whether an increase in lumpectomy rates would be associated with a concomitant increase in the rate of ipsilateral breast tumor recurrence, as well as to determine whether patients treated with such chemotherapy fared equally as well or better than those treated with standard postoperative chemotherapy.

Another consideration that led to the evaluation of preoperative chemotherapy related to the idea that if a correlation between the clinical and pathologic primary tumor response to preoperative chemotherapy and relapse-free survival could be unequivocally demonstrated, then response to such chemotherapy might be used both as a prognostic marker for outcome and as a guide in the selection of additional local-regional and systemic therapy for patients with operable breast cancer.[17,18]

RESULTS FROM NONRANDOMIZED TRIALS

Findings from several nonrandomized trials[16-20] have demonstrated that a variety of chemotherapeutic regimens administered preoperatively result in substantial rates of clinical response (47-85%) and in lesser rates of pathologic complete response (4-7%) (Table 1). Some of these studies have also shown that, when tumor size is reduced, more lumpectomies can be performed.

Findings from a study conducted by Jacquillat et al.[16] in 250 evaluable patients with stage I-IIIb carcinoma of the breast who received combined neoadjuvant and consolidation chemotherapy consisting of vinblastine (V), thiotepa (T), methotrexate (M), and fluorouracil (F) (VTMF) with or without doxorubicin [Adriamycin; (A)] followed by radiation therapy showed that primary chemotherapy induced tumor volume regression of more than 75% in 41% of the patients and complete clinical regression in 30%. At five years, breast preservation was 94%, and the cosmetic result was excellent or good in almost all of the patients.

Bonadonna et al.[17] administered preoperative chemotherapy to 33 patients in each of five groups (165 women), who were considered to be candidates for mastectomy because they had tumors with a diameter of at least 3 cm. One group received cyclophosphamide (C), methotrexate (M), and fluorouracil (F) (CMF) for three cycles; a second group received the same regimen (CMF) for four cycles. The third and fourth groups received FA (doxorubicin; Adriamycin) C (FAC), one for three cycles and the other for four cycles. The fifth group received FE (epirubicin) C (FEC) for three cycles.

Tumor shrinkage to less than 3 cm occurred in 127 patients (81%) after treatment with preoperative chemotherapy. This permitted breast-conserving surgery to be performed. Histopathologic complete remission was documented in seven patients. Degree of response was inversely proportional to initial tumor size, and frequency of response was greater in women with receptor-negative tumors.

Tubiana-Hulin et al.[18] treated a series of 150 stage IIIa breast cancer patients with AV (vincristine) CMF prior to surgery. An objective clinical tumor regression was observed in 47% of the patients, allowing for the performance of breast-conserving surgery in 35%. Clinical tumor regression was associated with freedom from distant metastases.

In a study involving 126 women with non-inflammatory operable breast cancer, who would otherwise have undergone modified radical mastectomy, Belembaogo et al.[19] administered induction chemotherapy, i.e., AVCF or AVCMF. Evidence of a decrease in tumor size was observed in 83% of patients. A greater response rate was observed in women with aneuploid or high S-phase tumors, particularly in women treated with methotrexate.

Finally, Smith et al.[20] reported that, in 84 patients who had operable breast cancer treated with primary chemotherapy (CMF, mitoxanthrone/ methotrexate/mitomycin C, or 5-FU/epirubicin/cisplatin), 69% of patients achieved an overall response with the first two regimens. Complete remissions were observed in 17% of these women and only 14% required mastectomy. With the third regimen, 84% of patients had an overall response; 58% of these women had complete remissions.

Although nonrandomized studies cannot evaluate the relative efficacy of preoperative vs. postoperative chemotherapy in terms of DFS and survival, they can provide useful information about the effect of preoperative chemotherapy on primary breast tumors and axillary-node involvement. Moreover, results from these studies can provide justification for the further evaluation of preoperative chemotherapy in randomized trials.

RESULTS FROM RANDOMIZED TRIALS

In 1991, Mauriac et al. of The Foundation Bergonie Bordeaux Group Trial reported on a randomized trial in 272 women with operable breast tumors larger than 3 cm.[21] Patients in the adjuvant therapy group (n = 138) were treated initially with modified radical mastectomy and adjuvant chemotherapy if they were either node positive or estrogen-receptor (ER) negative. Women in the neoadjuvant group were treated with chemotherapy followed by local-regional treatment that varied according to their response to chemotherapy. Thirty-two patients in the adjuvant therapy group did not receive adjuvant chemotherapy, and 44 patients in the neoadjuvant group who had a complete clinical response to chemotherapy did not undergo surgery but were treated with radiation therapy alone. After a median follow-up of 34 months, overall survival was better in women in the neoadjuvant chemotherapy group (p=0.04). However, these women also experienced an increased rate in the local recurrence of their tumors, a finding that could be explained by the fact that fewer of them underwent surgery. Because of the way in which the trial was designed, the question of whether preoperative chemotherapy was more effective than the same chemotherapy given in the adjuvant setting could not be adequately addressed. In fact, because more patients in the neoadjuvant group received chemotherapy, it is not surprising that an improvement in their overall survival was observed.

In 1994, Scholl et al.[22] from the Institute Curie reported on a randomized trial in which 414 premenopausal women with T2-T3, N0-N1, MO breast cancer were randomly assigned to receive either four cycles of neoadjuvant chemotherapy (CAF) followed by radiation therapy. Women with a persistent mass underwent surgery. Another group was treated with primary radiation therapy, with conservative surgery reserved for women with a persistent mass, followed by four cycles of the same chemotherapy. Of the 191 patients who could be evaluated in the preoperative chemotherapy group, 65% had an objective response after four cycles of therapy. With a median follow-up of 54 months, overall survival was significantly higher in the group that received neoadjuvant chemotherapy. No significant differences were observed in either DFS or local tumor recurrence. In accordance with the study design, 13% of the patients in the adjuvant group did not receive chemotherapy. These were women who had had surgery for an incomplete tumor regression after radiation therapy and who were found to be node negative on pathologic examination. The rate of breast conserving surgery was similar in both groups at the end of primary treatment. These findings can also be accounted for by the trial design, which created imbalances between the two groups in local as well as in systemic therapy, and should, thus, be viewed with skepticism.

In 1995, Powles et al. at the Royal Marsden Hospital reported findings from a small randomized trial in which the worth of systemic chemoendocrine therapy was evaluated as primary treatment before surgery in women with primary operable breast cancer.[23] Patients randomly assigned to neoadjuvant treatment received four cycles of chemotherapy for three months before surgery, followed by another four cycles of the same chemotherapy after surgery. Patients who were randomly assigned to adjuvant therapy received eight cycles of chemotherapy for six months after surgery. This trial did not directly compare adjuvant to neoadjuvant chemotherapy. Of the 212 randomized patients, 200 were able to be evaluated for response. The overall clinical response rate was 85%; the complete histologic response rate was 10%. There was a significant reduction in the number of mastectomies performed in women who received neoadjuvant therapy (13%), as compared with those who received adjuvant therapy. The median follow-up period of 28 months was too brief to allow for comparison of the relapse rate or survival outcome between the two groups.

In 1988, the National Surgical Adjuvant Breast and Bowel Project (NSABP) initiated a randomized trial, B18, in patients with operable breast cancer to compare preoperative vs. postoperative administration of adjuvant chemotherapy. After a diagnosis of breast cancer by fine needle aspiration (FNA) or core biopsy, patients were stratified according to age, clinical tumor size, and clinical nodal status and then were randomly assigned to receive either surgery (lumpectomy and axillary node dissection, or modified radical mastectomy) followed by four cycles of doxorubicin/cyclophosphamide (AC) chemotherapy every 21 days, or the same chemotherapy followed by surgery (Figure 1). Subsequent to completion of the adjuvant chemotherapy, all patients 50 years of age or older also received tamoxifen for five years. Patients who underwent lumpectomy also received postoperative radiation therapy, either after they recovered from surgery (the preoperative group), or after they completed all postoperative adjuvant chemotherapy (the postoperative group). The clinical size of breast and axillary tumors was determined before each of the four cycles of chemotherapy and before surgery. Between October 1988 and April 1993, 1523 women were randomized to the study: 760 in the preoperative group and 763 in the postoperative group. Results of the effect of preoperative chemotherapy on local-regional disease[24] demonstrated that 36% of patients achieved a clinical complete response and 44% a clinical partial response, for an overall clinical response rate of 80%. Stable disease was demonstrated in 17% of the patients, and 3% developed progressive disease. Tumor size and clinical nodal status were significant predictors of clinical complete response by multivariate analysis. Patients with small tumors and those with clinically positive nodes were more likely to achieve a clinical complete response. Of the latter, 26% were also found at the time of surgery to have a pathologic complete response, i.e., no residual tumor in either the lumpectomy or mastectomy specimen. In addition, 11% of the women who had a clinical complete response were found to have only noninvasive disease, i.e., ductal carcinoma in situ (DCIS) at the time of surgery.

There was clear evidence that preoperative chemotherapy resulted in axillary nodal downstaging. Whereas 43% of patients who received postoperative chemotherapy were found to have pathologically negative axillary nodes, 59% of patients who received preoperative chemotherapy were found to be node negative (p <0.001). Thus, there was a 37% increase in the incidence of pathologically negative nodes when chemotherapy was given before surgery. There was a highly significant correlation between tumor response to preoperative chemotherapy and pathologic nodal status. Seventy-four percent of patients with a complete clinical response had pathologically negative nodes, vs. 53% of patients with partial response, 50% of patients with stable disease, and 33% of patients with progressive disease.[25] Women who received preoperative chemotherapy were more likely to undergo a lumpectomy than were women who received postoperative chemotherapy (67% vs. 60%, p=0.002). This was particularly evident in women with tumors ≥5.1 cm in size (8% in the postoperative group vs. 22% in the preoperative group). After adjustment was made for clinical tumor size, a statistically significant correlation was observed between tumor response to preoperative chemotherapy and type of operation performed. Responding patients were more likely to have undergone a lumpectomy than were nonresponding patients (p=0.01).

When outcome results were compared, there was no significant difference in DFS, distant disease-free survival (DDFS), or overall survival between the group that received preoperative chemotherapy and the group that received postoperative chemotherapy.[26] For both groups through five years of follow-up, the DFS was 67% (p=0.99), the DDFS was 73% (p=0.70), and the overall survival was 80% (p=0.83). There was no significant difference between the two groups relative to the incidence and type of first events that occurred at local, regional, or distant sites. Although 5.8% of patients in the postoperative group and 7.9% in the preoperative group who underwent lumpectomy developed an ipsilateral breast tumor recurrence, this difference was not statistically significant. There was a significant correlation between clinical and pathologic response to preoperative chemotherapy and outcome. Patients who achieved a clinical complete response had a 76% DFS; the DFS was 64% for those who achieved a clinical partial response and 60% for those with stable disease (p=0.001). More important, among patients who achieved a clinical complete response, those who had a complete pathologic response had a significantly improved DFS and survival (84% vs. 87%, respectively) as compared with those who exhibited residual invasive carcinoma at the time of surgery (72% vs. 78%, respectively).

ADVANTAGES OF PREOPERATIVE CHEMOTHERAPY

Separating patients who received preoperative chemotherapy into groups according to their tumor response could provide a significant clinical advantage in their management. Because response to preoperative chemotherapy is a prognostic marker for DFS and survival, it can be used as an intermediate end point in determining the value of new regimens or for testing the effect of new drugs when these are administered after well-established regimens.[26] Because this intermediate end point can be achieved within weeks after a patient receives preoperative chemotherapy, new regimens could be evaluated and useful conclusions drawn without a five-to ten-year wait for follow-up, as is currently the case. Furthermore, with the availability of several new agents of demonstrated efficacy, breast cancer patients can be spared unnecessary treatment with ineffective regimens that do not translate into tumor response in the preoperative setting.[27]

Correlation of Prognostic Markers to Tumor Response

Evaluation of many of the proven, as well as putative, prognostic tumor markers, i.e., estrogen-receptor (ER), progesterone-receptor (PgR), ploidy, S-phase, erbB-2, p 53, and other tumor oncogenes and growth factors in material obtained by FNA or core biopsy could make possible the correlation of these markers with tumor response to preoperative chemotherapy, either individually or in combination. Conclusions could then be made relative to their prognostic value on DFS and overall survival and to their predictive value on tumor response without having to wait for several years of follow-up. With the primary tumor as the target, the manner in which new tumor markers are developed and evaluated could be altered. Moreover, it might eventually be possible to use such markers to identify patients with tumors undergoing clinical complete response who have a high likelihood of pathologic complete response and for whom further local therapy in the form of surgical resection and/or breast irradiation could be avoided.[27] Furthermore, serial monitoring of tumor marker changes while a patient is undergoing preoperative chemotherapy might provide biologic insight into the nature and function of these markers. Knowledge might also be obtained with regard to mechanisms of action of new chemotherapeutic regimens or treatment modalities.

Increase in Lumpectomy Rates

The potential for increasing the rates at which breast-conserving surgery is performed has provided most of the clinical justification for evaluating preoperative chemotherapy in patients with operable breast cancer. As indicated above, results from both nonrandomized and randomized studies have clearly demonstrated that the administration of preoperative chemotherapy results in higher lumpectomy rates. More important, in the NSABP B-18 study, this was accomplished without increasing the rates of ipsilateral breast tumor recurrence. With the development of more effective and clinically non-cross-resistant chemotherapeutic regimens that result in higher rates of clinical and pathologic tumor response, the potential exists for not only further increasing the rates of lumpectomy but also for eliminating surgical treatment altogether.

POTENTIAL DISADVANTAGES OF PREOPERATIVE CHEMOTHERAPY

False-Positive Fine Needle Aspiration (FNA)

Although, in the diagnosis of breast cancer, the rate of occurrence of a false-positive FNA is very low, invasive and noninvasive carcinoma cannot be readily differentiated by FNA, a potential weakness when it comes to using the technique for determining the presence of invasive carcinoma that should be treated with preoperative chemotherapy. A total of 651 patients in the postoperative chemotherapy group of the B-18 trial had their breast cancers diagnosed by FNA. Thirteen of these patients were found at surgery to have either benign pathology (two patients), lesions that did not require chemotherapy (seven patients with DCIS, one patient with adenoid cystic carcinoma, and two patients with cystosarcoma phyllodes), or lesions that did not require the specific chemotherapy that had been mandated in the protocol (one patient with lymphoma). Thus, the false-positive rate of FNA relative to diagnosis of cancer in the breast was 0.3%, but the false-positive rate relative to the selection of appropriate preoperative therapy was 2%. The development and widespread use of the core biopsy technique, which results in minimal tumor perturbation, has essentially eliminated the problem of a false-positive diagnosis. This technique is rapidly becoming the method of choice for the histologic diagnosis of breast cancer.

Overtreatment as the Result of Loss of
Prognostic Information from Pathologic Tumor Characteristics

One of the concerns surrounding the use of preoperative chemotherapy relates to the unnecessary treatment of some patients who may not need adjuvant chemotherapy based on pathologic tumor and nodal characteristics that are not available before surgery. The use of core needle biopsy rather than FNA provides enough material for the evaluation of most of the important prognostic and predictive tumor markers, e.g., ER/PgR, erbB-2, ploidy, and S-phase. Furthermore, with the demonstration of a benefit from adjuvant chemotherapy in both node-positive as well as node-negative breast cancer patients,[2,28] knowledge of pathologic nodal status is usually not a requirement when the decision about whether or not to use adjuvant chemotherapy is made, except in patients with small tumors (<1 cm), in whom a small benefit from chemotherapy may not justify its use, and in patients with other comorbid conditions, in whom the use of chemotherapy might not be in their best interest. Currently available information about the benefit from adjuvant chemotherapy and current biopsy techniques have facilitated decision making with regard to the need for adjuvant chemotherapy in the majority of breast cancer patients with operable disease before surgical extirpation of their tumor and have, thus, permitted consideration of the use of preoperative chemotherapy.

Issues Related to Cost and Convenience

Although, in terms of cost, there is no difference between whether chemotherapy is used in either the preoperative or the postoperative settings, additional expense, as well as inconvenience, may be encountered in the preoperative setting as a result of additional visits to the surgeon during chemotherapy for the purpose of monitoring response and operability and the additional cost of mammograms and procedures such as wire localization, which is used if a tumor is nonpalpable. However, when considered relative to the potential benefit of preserving the breast and obtaining information that can be used for patient management, these issues are minor.

SURGICAL CONSIDERATIONS

Several surgical considerations need to be taken into account in a patient who receives preoperative chemotherapy. The first relates to the ability to identify the exact tumor location in those instances in which a complete clinical response has occurred. In the majority of such cases, residual mammographic abnormalities remain; this makes wire localization and, thus, tumor removal possible. However, some patients with a clinical complete response show no evidence of tumor on mammographic evaluation. In such cases, the patient should be closely monitored and the area of mammographic abnormality marked, before its disappearance, with a titanium clip for future identification. In cases where the primary tumor is poorly visible mammographically because of dense breast parenchyma, the placement of the surgical clip should precede initiation of preoperative chemotherapy. Clip placement is crucial in cases of pathologic complete response, because it allows pathologists to focus their attention on that area in the search for residual tumor. Moreover, in patients with pathologic complete response who undergo lumpectomy, placement of the clip ensures that the area in which the tumor was previously located has been accurately identified and that residual tumor is not left behind after removal of the primary tumor.

The second consideration relates to the amount of breast tissue that needs to be removed during lumpectomy in responding patients. In this circumstance, the question arises as to whether the tissue removal should account for the original tumor size or whether it should be limited to an adequate margin around the residual tumor after chemotherapy. The answer to this question depends on the original tumor configuration, i.e., on whether it is well-circumscribed or irregular with projections, on the presence or absence of suspicious microcalcifications that would indicate an extensive intraductal component, and on the size of the breast and the potential for compromise of the cosmetic outcome if lumpectomy based on the original tumor size were to be performed. It is reasonable to plan the lumpectomy on the basis of the residual tumor size after chemotherapy; however, the status of the surgical margins must be carefully assessed and the surgeon must be prepared to perform additional resection if, on pathologic evaluation, the margins are found to have been compromised.

CURRENT STATUS AND FUTURE DIRECTIONS

The role of preoperative chemotherapy in the treatment of operable breast cancer continues to evolve. In view of the findings from NSABP B-18, such treatment can be used interchangeably with adjuvant chemotherapy and would be most appropriate in patients who would prefer to preserve their breasts but who have tumors too large for breast-conserving surgery. Another potential advantage of preoperative chemotherapy is that, unlike with postoperative chemotherapy, clinical and pathologic tumor response can be used not only as prognostic factors for outcome but also as guidelines for further local-regional and systemic therapy.

The development of taxanes, a new class of chemotherapeutic agents with a novel mechanism of action, and the demonstration of their significant antitumor activity in patients with advanced breast cancer provide the opportunity for further evaluation of some of the concepts that have emerged from the first generation of trials of preoperative chemotherapy. In 1995, the NSABP implemented B-27, a randomized trial being conducted to determine whether the preoperative or postoperative administration of docetaxel after preoperative doxorubicin/cyclophosphamide (AC) therapy will prolong DFS and overall survival to a greater extent than will four courses of preoperative AC therapy alone (Figure 2).[29,30] Equally important are the secondary aims of this trial, which are to determine whether the administration of preoperative docetaxel after preoperative AC therapy will further increase the clinical and pathologic response rates of primary breast tumors and whether it will result in further axillary nodal downstaging and, thus, an increase in the rates at which lumpectomies are performed. A comparison of the administration of postoperative docetaxel after preoperative AC therapy to preoperative AC alone will identify whether any improvement in DFS and/or overall survival will occur uniformly or in subgroups of patients, i.e., in patients with residual positive nodes. Two ancillary studies to the B-27 trial are attempting to evaluate serum and tumor biomarkers as they relate to outcome and response to preoperative AC therapy or to chemotherapy with docetaxel. The first trial (B-27.1) has been designed to evaluate the worth of serum erbB-2 extracellular domain (ECD) and serum anti-erbB-2 and antibodies in predicting response to preoperative chemotherapy and long-term outcome in patients randomized to B-27. In addition, obtaining serum at specified times, i.e., before administration and after completion of preoperative chemotherapy, after surgery, one year after randomization, and at the time of tumor recurrence will enable investigators to evaluate whether changes in the levels of erbB-2 ECD and anti-erbB-2 antibodies are induced by chemotherapy or are associated with tumor recurrence. The second trial (B-27.2) has been designed to evaluate whether tumor biomarkers obtained by FNA or core biopsy can be used to predict response to preoperative chemotherapy and long-term outcome in B-27 patients. Another aim of B-27.2 is to determine whether preoperative chemotherapy results in changes in tumor biomarker expression and whether these changes can be correlated with tumor response and long-term outcome. The biomarkers being evaluated are nuclear grade, ER and PgR receptors, proliferation markers, p53, erbB-2 oncoprotein, P-glycoprotein, and bcl-2.

Two potential lines of investigation can be followed relative to the future development of studies with neoadjuvant chemotherapy. The first approach relates to the evaluation of more effective chemotherapy regimens in the neoadjuvant setting, with the intent of further reducing the extent of local treatment in the breast and axilla. In the breast, this approach would necessitate the use of tumor biomarkers to predict which patients with clinical complete response are also more likely to have a pathologic complete response. Core biopsies of the area of the tumor bed may be required to confirm a pathologic complete response. Similarly, in the axilla, the sentinel-node biopsy technique may permit the identification of sentinel-node-negative patients who would not need further axillary dissection should this procedure be validated in randomized trials, in particular, in patients who receive preoperative chemotherapy. The second approach relates to the use of primary tumor response to chemotherapy as in vivo chemosensitivity assay so that the most appropriate chemotherapy regimens can be administered and so that the patient does not have to undergo administration of chemotherapy that does not have any effect on the tumor.

SUMMARY

In the NSABP B-18 study, it was demonstrated that, in patients with operable breast cancer, the administration of preoperative and postoperative chemotherapy resulted in similar DFS and overall survival outcomes. In addition, preoperative chemotherapy resulted in high clinical response rates but in low rates of pathologic response in the breast. Axillary nodal downstaging was convincingly demonstrated. In addition, it was also demonstrated in B-18, as well as in other studies, that there was an increase in breast conservation rates after the administration of preoperative chemotherapy. The role of preoperative chemotherapy for operable breast cancer continues to be evaluated in randomized trials, which have the potential of providing further insight into the biologic and clinical questions relative to the timing of adjuvant therapy for the disease.

REFERENCES

1. Fisher B: Laboratory and clinical research in breast cancer—a personal adventure: the David A. Karnofsky Memorial Lecture. Cancer Res; 40:3863-3874, 1980.
2. Early Breast Cancer Trialists' Collaborative Group: Effects of radiotherapy and surgery in early breast cancer: an overview of the randomized trials. N Eng J Med; 333:1444-1455, 1995.
3. Early Breast Cancer Trialists' Collaborative Group: Systemic treatment of early breast cancer by hormonal, cytoxic, or immune therapy: 133 randomised trials involving 31,000 recurrences and 24,000 deaths among 75,000 women. Lancet; 339:1-15 (Part 1), 71-85 (Part 2), 1992.
4. Skipper HE: Kinetics of mammary tumor cell growth and implications for therapy. Cancer; 28:1479-1499, 1971.
5. Goldie JH and Coldman AJ: A mathematical model for relating the drug sensitivity of tumors to their spontaneous mutation rate. Cancer Treat Rep; 63:1727-1733, 1979.
6. Gunduz N, Fisher B, Saffer EA: Effect of surgical removal on the growth and kinetics of residual tumor. Cancer Res; 39:3861-3865, 1979.
7. Fisher B, Gunduz N, and Saffer EA: Influence of the interval between primary tumor removal and chemotherapy of kinetics and growth of metastases. Cancer Res; 43:1488-1492, 1983.
8. Rosen G: Preoperative chemotherapy for osteogenic sarcoma. Cancer; 49:1221-1230, 1982.
9. Schuller DE: Preoperative reductive chemotherapy for locally advanced carcinoma of the oral activity, oropharynx, and hypopharynx. Cancer; 51:15-19, 1983.
10. Leichman L, Steiger Z, Seydel HG, et al: Preoperative chemotherapy and radiation therapy for patients with cancer of the esophagus: a potentially curative approach. J Clin Oncol; 2:75-79, 1984.
11. Perloff M, Lesnick J: Chemotherapy before and after mastectomy in Stage III breast cancer. Arch Surg; 117:879-881, 1982.
12. Schick P, Goodstein J, Moor J, et al: Preoperative chemotherapy followed by mastectomy for locally advanced breast cancer. J Surg Oncol; 22:278-282, 1983.
13. Sorace RA, Bagley CS, Lichter AS, et al: The management of nonmetastatic locally advanced breast cancer using primary induction chemotherapy with hormonal synchronization followed by radiation therapy with or without debulking surgery. World J Surg; 9:775-785, 1985.
14. Fisher B, Redmond C, Poisson R, et al: Eight-year results of a randomized clinical trial comparing mastectomy and lumpectomy with or without

irradiation in the treatment of breast cancer. N Engl J Med; 320:820-828, 1989.

15. Fisher B, Anderson S, Redmond C, et al: Reanalysis and results after 12-year follow-up in a randomized clinical trial comparing total mastectomy with lumpectomy with or without irradiation in the treatment of breast cancer. N Engl J Med; 333:1456-1461, 1995.

16. Jacquillat C, Weil M, Baillet F, et al: Results of neoadjuvant chemotherapy and radiation therapy in breast conserving treatment of 250 patients with all stages of infiltrative breast cancer. Cancer; 66:119-129, 1990.

17. Bonadonna G, Veronesi U, Brambilla C, et al: Primary chemotherapy to avoid mastectomy in tumors with diameters of three centimeters or more. J Natl Cancer Inst; 82:1539-1545, 1990.

18. Tubiana-Hulin M, Malek M, Briffod M, et al: Preoperative chemotherapy of operable breast cancer (stage IIIA). Prognostic factors of distant recurrence. Eur J Cancer; Vol. 29A, Suppl. 6:S76 (#391), 1993.

19. Belembaogo E, Feillel V, Chollet P, et al: Neoadjuvant chemotherapy in 126 operable breast cancers. Eur J Cancer; Vol. 28A, 4/5:896-900, 1992.

20. Smith IE, Jones AL, O'Brien MER, et al: Primary medical (neo-adjuvant) chemotherapy for operable breast cancer. Eur J Cancer; Vol. 29A, 12:1796-1799, 1993.

21. Mauriac L, Durand M, Avril A, Dilhuydy J-M: Effects on primary chemotherapy in conservative treatment of breast cancer patients with operable tumors larger than 3 cm. Ann Oncol; 2:347-354, 1991.

22. Scholl SM, Fourquet A, Asselain B, et al: Neoadjuvant versus adjuvant chemotherapy in premenopausal patients with tumours considered too large for breast conserving surgery: preliminary results of a randomized trial: S6. Eur J Cancer; 30:645-652, 1994.

23. Powles TJ, Hickish TF, Makris A, et al: Randomized trial of chemoendocrine therapy started before or after surgery for treatment of primary breast cancer. J Clin Oncol; 13:547-552, 1995.

24. Fisher B, Brown A, Mamounas E, et al: Effect of preoperative chemotherapy of local-regional disease in women with operable breast cancer: findings from National Surgical Adjuvant Breast and Bowel Project B-18. J Clin Oncol; 15:2483-2493, 1997.

25. Fisher B, Rockette H, Robidoux A, et al: Effect of preoperative therapy for breast cancer (BC) on local-regional disease: First report of NSABP B-18. Proc Am Soc Clin Oncol; 13:64, 1994 (abstr. 57).

26. Fisher B, Bryant J, Wolmark N, et al: Effect of preoperative chemotherapy on the outcome of women with operable breast cancer. J Clin Oncol; 16:2672-2685, 1998.

27. Fisher B, Mamounas EP: Preoperative chemotherapy: a model for studying the biology and therapy of primary breast cancer. J Clin Oncol; 13:537-540, 1995.

28. Fisher B, Dignam J, Wolmark N, et al: Tamoxifen and chemotherapy for lymph node-negative, estrogen receptor-positive breast cancer. J Natl Cancer Inst; 89:1673-1682, 1997.

29. Mamounas EP: NSABP Protocol B-27: preoperative doxorubicin plus cyclophosphamide followed by preoperative or postoperative docetaxel. Oncology; Suppl. 6:37-40, 1997.

30. Mamounas EP: Overview of National Surgical Adjuvant Breast Project neoadjuvant chemotherapy studies. Semin Oncol; 25 (Suppl 3):31-35, 1998.

Table 1. Nonrandomized Trials of Preoperative Chemotherapy for Operable Breast Cancer

Trial	Number of Evaluable Patients	Tumor Stage/Size	Regimen	Clinical Complete Response %	Clinical Partial Response %	Pathologic Complete Response %	Overall Response %
Jacquillat[16]	250	I-IIIB	VTMF ± A	30	41*	N/A†	71
Bonadonna[17]	161	3 cm	CMF x 3-4 CAF x 3-4 FEC x 3	17	60	4	77
Tubiana-Hulin[18]	150	IIIA	AVCMF	—	—	—	47
Belembaogo[19]	124	Operable	AVCF/ AVCMF	36	49	7‡	85
Smith[20]	84	Large, operable	CMF MMM FEC	17 58	52 26	— —	69 84

* Greater than 75% reduction.
† Patients underwent radiotherapy after chemotherapy.
‡ In 83 patients who underwent surgery

Figure 1

NSABP B-18 SCHEMA

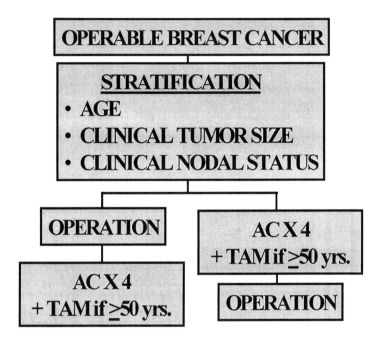

Figure 2

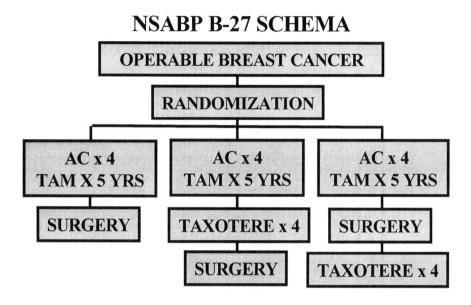

8

Overview of Randomized Trials of Systemic Adjuvant Therapy

Peter M. Ravdin, MD
Associate Professor of Medicine
University of Texas Health Science Center at San Antonio

INTRODUCTION

The most influential analyses of the effectiveness of systemic adjuvant therapy of breast cancer are the 3 overview meta-analyses performed at Oxford and published in 1988[1], 1992[2], and 1998[3]. These meta-analyses are a collaborative effort dependent on pooling of data by trialists of nearly all the randomized clinical trials of systemic adjuvant therapies. The major questions that were addressed by these Overview analyses were:

1) Is systemic adjuvant therapy of breast cancer effective?

2) Are there subsets of patients in whom given adjuvant therapies are particularly effective?

3) How effective is the current adjuvant therapy?

These analyses have been particularly influential because they have included very large number of patients giving them great statistical power. They also have brought some sense and order to understanding the massive literature reporting the dozens of trials evaluating the effectiveness of adjuvant therapy. These Overview analyses have the potential weakness of obscuring important differences in the design of trials (i.e., dose, duration, scheduling).

Therefore these analyses are useful benchmark evaluations of the average effectiveness of systemic adjuvant therapies.

HOW ARE THE OVERVIEW RESULTS REPORTED?

Proportional Risk Reductions

It is important to understand the nature of the estimates of the effectiveness of proportional risk reductions given in the Overview analysis. Proportional risk reductions can be viewed as the percentage of negative outcomes that were avoided because a systemic adjuvant therapy was used. For example let us examine a scenario where a patient has a 25% risk of relapse if they do not receive therapy, and they subsequently receive a systemic adjuvant therapy that provides a 40% proportional risk reduction of recurrence. In a simplistic way, this means that if the risk of a negative event (25%) is multiplied by the proportional risk reduction provided by the adjuvant therapy (40%), an absolute reduction in the odds of relapse of 10% is provided to the patient. The risk of relapse is reduced from 25% to 15% in this example for patients receiving adjuvant systemic therapy. This is the method commonly used in the clinic to calculate proportional risk reductions supplied by the Overview analyses. Although this method is useful in practice, it needs to be recognized that it gives fairly inaccurate approximation for patients that have risk of negative outcomes of 50% or greater.

An important but subtle fact is that the Overview analysis actually provides proportional risk reductions for the *annual* risk of a negative event (recurrence or death). This annual risk *compounds* to give the risk at some future time. For a patient with a 10-year risk of a negative event of 60%, the actual annual risk is about 8.8%. This leads to a year-by-year *cumulative* estimate of a negative outcome for years 1 to 10 of 8.8, 16.7, 24.0, 30.7, 36.8, 42.3, 47.3, 52.0, 56.2 and 60.0%, respectively.

If the annual risk is reduced by a proportional 20% by an adjuvant therapy regimen, then the resulting risks would be 8.8% x 0.8 giving the result of a 7% annual risk. This leads to a year-by-year cumulative estimate of a negative outcome in years 1 to 10 of 7.0, 13.5, 19.6, 25.2, 30.4, 35.3, 39.9, 44.1, 48.0, and 51.6%, respectively. This leads to an estimated change of the risk of negative outcome from 60% with no treatment to 51.6% for patients receiving an adjuvant therapy conveying a 20% proportional risk reduction in the annual hazard. The net absolute benefit is therefore 8% rather than the 12% that the simpler method would estimate.

THE HISTORICAL IMPACT OF THE
1988 AND 1992 OVERVIEWS

The first two Overview analyses helped define the standard of care, and to define the questions to be addressed by clinical trials. The size of these analyses can be seen in the following table.

Year of Analysis		Trials (n=)	Patients (n=)
1988φ	Tamoxifen	28	16,513
	Chemotherapy	31	9,069
1992φ	Tamoxifen	40	29,892
	Chemotherapy	44	18,403

φ The duration of follow-up for the 1988 analysis was ~5 years, and for the 1992 analysis was ~ 10 years.

The proportional risk reductions for *mortality* estimated by these two Overview analysis were:

Proportional Risk Reduction Estimates for Mortality in 1988 and 1992

1988 Overview	Subset by nodal status	% Proportional Risk Reduction (standard error) [φ]	
		For Tamoxifen	For Polychemotherapy
Premenopausal	Any	1 (9)	26 (7)
Postmenopausal	Any	23 (4)	8 (6)
1992 Overview			
Premenopausal	Any	6 (5)	27 (6)
	Node Negative	19 (12)	6 (13)
	Node Positive	5 (5)	30 (6)
Postmenopausal	Any	20 (2)	14 (5)
	Node Negative	16 (5)	23 (11)
	Node Positive	22 (3)	11 (4)

[φ] Two times the SE defines the ~ limits of the 95% confidence interval.

    The 1988 analysis included data from trials conducted in the 1970's and early 1980's. The studies of the effectiveness of adjuvant tamoxifen (TAM) showed a clear benefit in postmenopausal women but raised questions as to its effectiveness in premenopausal women. The 1988 analysis also showed clear benefit for adjuvant systemic polychemotherapy (C) in premenopausal women but left open the questions as to whether adjuvant chemotherapy was effective in postmenopausal women.

    There were however some important limitations of the 1988 analysis. Many of the studies evaluating tamoxifen used durations of tamoxifen of 2 years of less, durations that we recognize as inadequate today. For the analysis of the effectiveness of adjuvant polychemotherapy the statistical power was insufficient to address whether there was some degree of benefit in postmenopausal women. The statistical power of this Overview analysis was insufficient to address the question of whether both node negative (NN) and node positive (NP) subsets benefited from therapy, although the trends in the data suggested no major differences in proportional risk reductions on the basis of nodal status. Because estrogen receptor (ER) determinations were available on fewer than half the patients in the tamoxifen trials, the 1988 Overview analysis was not able to make a clear statement as to whether ER was a strong predictor of the benefit of adjuvant tamoxifen.

The second Overview analysis in 1992 had greater statistical power because it included a greater number of patients followed for a longer time. This second analysis confirmed the value of tamoxifen in postmenopausal patients, with the suggestion that it was of less benefit in premenopausal patients. This analysis also suggested that ER expression was a predictor of the amount of benefit derived from adjuvant tamoxifen, but the analysis left open the question as to whether ER poor or negative patients obtained some lesser degree of benefit. The second Overview analysis was able to show that the benefit of tamoxifen did occur in both NN and NP patients. The results of the 1992 analysis of adjuvant polychemotherapy differed in important ways from the 1988 analysis. It was now clear that both pre- and postmenopausal women benefited from adjuvant polychemotherapy, although the degree of benefit was clearly less in the postmenopausal patients.

Thus the 1988 and 1992 Overview analyses set the stage for future analyses. They established the precedent for collaborative pooling of data from many trials, and they showed in broad strokes in which patients systemic therapies were particularly effective. They showed that at best the effectiveness of these therapies was modest and that clearly there was a need for further studies and new ideas. Finally they set the stage for further Overview analyses that were necessary to more clearly show which subsets of patients benefited from adjuvant therapy. The enormous database also allowed investigators to determine the optimal duration of tamoxifen therapy and the contribution of anthracyclines in chemotherapy programs.

1998 OVERVIEW OF THE EFFECTIVENESS OF ADJUVANT TAMOXIFEN

Introduction

The most recent Overview analysis is perhaps the most valuable of the three for a number of reasons:

(1) This meta-analysis now includes several trials in which patients were randomized to receive 5 years of tamoxifen. In the past, the analyses were dominated by the results of trials in which tamoxifen was given for 2 years or less. Since that time, the results from a large randomized trial of different

tamoxifen durations suggest that the appropriate duration of tamoxifen therapy is 5 years, and that shorter durations were inferior[5].

(2) In the past, proportional risk reductions were reported for recurrence, and also for combined recurrence and mortality. It was not possible to define what the impact of adjuvant therapy was on overall mortality. The present analysis is reported with 2 major endpoints; reduction in recurrence, and reduction in mortality.

(3) There is now more that 10 years of follow-up on many trials, giving the 1998 analysis more statistical power.

The overall conclusion of the most recent Overview analysis is that for women with ER-positive (or unknown and probably positive) early breast cancer, adjuvant tamoxifen causes substantial reductions in risk of recurrence and death, irrespective of nodal status, age or menopausal status, and whether the patient received chemotherapy.

The central questions addressed by the Overview analysis were:

How long should Tamoxifen be given?

5 years appears superior to shorter durations.
Although the optimal duration of tamoxifen cannot be formally assessed in trials in which there was not a head-to-head comparison of different tamoxifen durations, it can be inferred indirectly from the results of the Overview analysis shown in Table 1. All durations of tamoxifen clearly benefit patients, but longer durations conferred more benefit. This is consistent with the Swedish trial, which showed that 5 years of adjuvant tamoxifen was superior to 2 years.[5] The results of the NSABP B-14 trial suggested that continuation of adjuvant tamoxifen beyond 5 years did not confer any additional benefit[6]. Therefore at this time the widely accepted standard of care for adjuvant tamoxifen duration is 5 years, and this is supported by the current Overview analysis.

Proportional Risk Reductions
Achieved by Tamoxifen of Different Durations

	$n = ^\nabla$	% Proportional Risk Reduction (standard error) $^\phi$	
Duration of Tamoxifen		Recurrence	Death
About 1 year	4543/4585	18 (3)	10 (3)
About 2 years	9838/9784	25 (2)	15 (2)
3 or more years*	4184/4165	42 (3)	22 (4)

* Median duration 5 years
$^\nabla$ Number of patients in the trials who received tamoxifen vs the number who did not.
$^\phi$ Two times the SE defines the ~ limits of the 95% confidence interval.

Should Tamoxifen be given to ER-negative patients?

Although this question is open to further research, tamoxifen therapy for ER-negative patients is not strongly supported by the current Overview analysis.
The question of whether estrogen receptor negative patients benefit from tamoxifen was addressed by the Overview analysis. There was a clear benefit conferred by tamoxifen in ER-positive patients, and no statistically significant benefit seen in the ER-poor patients. If there is a benefit conferred by tamoxifen in ER-negative patients it is small.

Proportional Risk Reduction of Adverse Outcome at 10 Years Follow-up*
Does Estrogen Receptor Status Make A Difference?

		% Proportional Risk Reduction (standard error)	
Estrogen Receptor Level	N=	Recurrence	Death
ER-poor	446/476	6 (11)	-3 (11)
ER-unknown	772/786	37 (8)	21 (9)
ER-positive #	2966/2903	50 (4)	28 (5)

* For patients receiving tamoxifen for a median duration 5 years
# Defined a $\geq$ 10 fentomoles of ER per mg of cytosol if quantitated, otherwise accepted as reported

The Overview analysis did examine whether tamoxifen was beneficial in patients with very high levels of ER ($\geq$ 100 fentomoles of ER/mg cytosol protein) as compared to patients with lower levels of ER (10–99 fentomoles of ER/mg cytosol protein).

Proportional Risk Reduction of Adverse Outcome at 10 Years Follow-up*
Does Estrogen Receptor Level Make A Difference?

Estrogen Receptor Level	N=	% Proportional Risk Reduction (standard error)	
		Recurrence	Death
ER (10-99 fm/mg)	Not given	43 (5)	23 (6)
ER (> 100 fm/mg)	Not given	60 (6)	36 (7)

* For patients receiving tamoxifen for a median duration 5 years

The Overview analysis also examined whether the use of progesterone receptor (PR) determinations allowed refinement of the estimates of benefit. This analysis was not ideal, because PR information was available on fewer of the patients, and because there were very few patients in certain subsets (ER negative, PR-positive). Thus the analysis was restricted to patients who were ER-positive and PR-negative. These patients seemed to benefit to a similar degree to ER-positive patients overall with reductions in the risk of recurrence of 46% ($\pm$ 9) and mortality of 28% ($\pm$ 11).

Does Tamoxifen benefit both premenopausal and postmenopausal patients?

Yes.
Overall the effectiveness of tamoxifen did not seem to be strongly modulated by age. The one subset that did not seem to benefit as much included those patients 50-59 years of age. No comment was made about this observation in the Overview analysis. Also, patients 50-59 years of age did not seem to experience a statistically significant outcome different than those overall (who had a 47% and a 26% proportional risk reduction for recurrence or death). Thus the low degree of mortality reduction seen for 50-59 year old women in the trials with 5 years of tamoxifen might be interpreted as an artifact caused by the play of chance (some such deviations from the expected occur when multiple subset analyses are done).

Proportional Risk Reduction of Adverse Outcome at 10 Years Follow-Up Effects of Patient Age on the Effectiveness of Tamoxifen

| Age (years) | N= | % Proportional Risk Reduction (standard error) | |
		Recurrence	Death
< 50	661/666	45 (8)	32 (10)
50-59	1285/1251	37 (6)	11 (8)
60-69	1606/1568	54 (5)	33 (6)
≥ 70	186/204	54 (13)	34 (13)

For patients receiving tamoxifen for a median duration 5 years, who were ER positive or ER unknown

Age is more reliably recorded than menopausal status, and thus analyses were done on the basis of age rather than menopausal status. Women aged 40-49 years and 50-59 years were further subdivided by menopausal status, and that subdivision did not affect age-specific results.

Does Tamoxifen confer benefit for both Node Negative (NN) and Node Positive (NP) patients?

Yes.
This question was addressed in the 1998 meta-analysis. The degree of benefit in terms of proportional risk reduction is the same in NN and NP patients.

Proportional Risk Reduction of Adverse Outcome at 10 Years Follow-Up Effects of Node Status

| Nodal Status | N= | % Proportional Risk Reduction (standard error) | |
		Recurrence	Death
Node negative	2611/2606	49 (4)	25 (5)
Node positive	1127/1083	43 (5)	28 (6)

For patients receiving tamoxifen for a median duration 5 years, who were ER positive or ER unknown

The absolute net benefit of tamoxifen would be expected to be less for patients with NN disease because in patients with a lower risk of recurrence and death the proportional risk reduction afforded by adjuvant tamoxifen will be less. This effect was obvious for absolute mortality reduction in both NN and NP patients.

Absolute Reduction of Adverse Outcome at 10 Years Follow-Up Effects of Nodal Status

		% Absolute Risk Reduction	
Nodal Status	N=	Recurrence	Death
Node negative	2611/2606	15%	6%
Node positive	1127/1083	15%	11%

For patients receiving tamoxifen for a median duration 5 years, who were ER positive or ER unknown

Do patients who receive adjuvant chemotherapy benefit from the addition of adjuvant tamoxifen?

Yes.

The Overview analysis found that adjuvant chemotherapy plus 5 years of tamoxifen was substantially better that chemotherapy alone. The 95% confidence intervals overlap for the proportional benefits of chemotherapy with and without tamoxifen, so it can not be stated that tamoxifen is actually more effective in women that received chemotherapy (and this was not the case for trials in which women received 1 or 2 years of adjuvant tamoxifen). Nonetheless it is clear that tamoxifen does not appear in any way less effective in women who received adjuvant chemotherapy.

Absolute Reduction of Adverse Outcome at 10 Years Follow-Up Effects of Concurrent Chemotherapy on Whether Tamoxifen is Effective

		% Proportional Risk Reduction (standard error)	
Trial Design	N=	Recurrence	Death
Tam vs Nil	3253/3229	46 (4)	22 (5)
Tam + C vs C	485/460	52 (8)	47 (9)

For patients receiving tamoxifen for a median duration 5 years, who were ER positive or ER unknown

Unfortunately the relatively low numbers of patients in the Tam + C versus C trials does not allow statistically reliable statements to be made about whether the additional benefit of tamoxifen was equally large in both pre- and postmenopausal women. The analysis shown below suggests that there are not major differences, but because of large standard errors the interaction of age plus chemotherapy on efficacy is still uncertain; however, it does not appear greatly different. The results of the soon to be reported trials such as Intergroup 0100 (comparing CMF with CAF, with and without tamoxifen) may help clarify this question. This result is also consistent with the results of the meta-analysis of adjuvant oophorectomy trials in which adjuvant oophorectomy clearly added to the effectiveness of adjuvant chemotherapy.[7]

Absolute Reduction of Adverse Outcome at 10 Years Follow-Up
Effects of Concurrent Chemotherapy and Age on
Whether Tamoxifen is Effective

Trial Design	N=	% Proportional Risk Reduction (standard error)	
		Recurrence	Death
Tam vs Nil <50 yr	not given	47 (8)	30 (12)
Tam vs Nil ≥50 yr	not given	45 (4)	20 (5)
Tam + C vs C <50 yr	not given	40 (19)	39 (22)
Tam + C vs C ≥50 yr	not given	54 (8)	49 (10)

For patients receiving tamoxifen for a median duration 5 years, who were ER positive or ER unknown

Is tamoxifen safe, and does it confer net health benefits?

Risk of endometrial cancer is increased.
Risk of second primary breast cancer is reduced ~40% over the next decade.
There is no effect on net non-breast cancer related mortality.
The Overview analysis allows the magnitude of the potential risks and benefits of tamoxifen to be assessed. The data from the Overview analysis

suggest that the excess risk of endometrial cancer is approximately 1%, but that the excess risk of death due to endometrial cancer was more modest at ~0.2%. This is consistent with previous reviews addressing this concern[8].

On the basis of an apparent excess of colorectal cancer in a subset of adjuvant trials the question of whether tamoxifen may increase colorectal cancer was analyzed. In the Overview analysis, there is not an excess of colorectal cancer in patients receiving tamoxifen.

The Overview analysis published in 1992 suggested that there might be a reduction of cardiovascular mortality due to tamoxifen. This reduction might be expected on the basis on favorable effects of tamoxifen on HDL/LDL ratios and total cholesterol[9]. However, this effect was not observed in the 1998 Overview analysis, although modest effects on cardiovascular mortality were not excluded. All cause mortality (of which cardiovascular mortality was a major component) was not affected by tamoxifen.

An approximate 40% reduction in contralateral breast cancer was again documented in patients getting 5 years of tamoxifen.

Absolute Reduction of Adverse Outcome at
Approximately 10 Years Follow-Up

	10 year risk per 1,000 Patients		Significant Difference?
	Tamoxifen	Control	
Endometrial Cancer Incidence	11	3	Yes
Endometrial Cancer Mortality	2	0	Yes
Colorectal Cancer Incidence	9	7	No
Non-Breast or Endometrial Cancer Mortality	59	58	No
Contralateral breast cancer incidence	26	47	Yes

For patients receiving tamoxifen for a median duration 5 years

SUMMARY

The strongest conclusion of the 1998 Overview analysis is that if a patient's tumor is ER-positive, then adjuvant tamoxifen administered for 5 years should produce benefits, largely irrespective of age or menopausal status, nodal status, or prior adjuvant chemotherapy. It was noted however that these were proportional benefits, and the absolute amount of benefit would depend on the baseline risk of the patient, and might be relatively small in patients with small localized tumors of good histological grade.

Overall the 1998 Overview strongly supported the use of adjuvant tamoxifen therapy.

THE 1998 OVERVIEW ANALYSIS OF RANDOMIZED ADJUVANT CHEMOTHERAPY TRIALS

Introduction

The 1998 Overview analysis reports the effects of polychemotherapy in randomized adjuvant trials. This is the third such Overview published with earlier analyses published in 1981 and 1992. The most recent Overview analyses are perhaps the most valuable of the three for a number of reasons.

(1) There is now more than 10 years of follow-up on many trials, giving the 1998 Overview analysis more statistical power. The analysis of chemotherapy versus no chemotherapy is based on 47 trials involving 17,723 patients. Analysis of longer versus shorter chemotherapy is based on 11 trials involving 6,104 patients. Analysis of anthracycline-containing regimens versus non-anthracycline (CMF) based regimens is based on 11 trials involving 5,942 patients.

(2) The presentation of the analysis has changed in a way to make it more useful to the clinician. In the past the proportional risk reductions were reported for recurrence, and also for recurrence and mortality combined. This second endpoint is not as easily interpretable as mortality. The present analysis is reported with 2 major endpoints: reduction in recurrence, and reduction in mortality.

Recurrence was defined as the first reappearance or breast cancer at any site. Deaths from an unknown cause were included as deaths due to breast cancer unless it was specifically stated that breast cancer was not the cause.

The questions addressed by the meta-analysis included:

Is polychemotherapy effective?

Yes. Overall results show that adjuvant polychemotherapy reduces the risk of both recurrence and death.

The results of the 1998 Overview analysis show a statistically significant benefit afforded by several months of polychemotherapy for the average patient participating in these trials (Table 1). This benefit was reflected in a reduced risk of recurrence and mortality. There was no statistically significant difference in the degree of benefit in the categories of polychemotherapy or between the separate individual trials.

Table 1: Proportional Risk Reduction of Adverse Outcome For Patients Treated with Polychemotherapy: Overall Effectiveness

	N=[*]	% Proportional Risk Reduction (standard error)[φ]	
Regimen		Recurrence	Death
CMF	4103/4047	24 (3)	14 (4)
CMF + extra cytotoxics	1622/1596	20 (2)	15 (5)
Other polychemotherapy	3701/3719	25 (4)	17 (4)
Average Polychemotherapy	9426/9362	24 (2)	15 (2)

[*] Number of patients in the trials who received polychemotherapy vs the number who did not.

[φ] Two times the SE defines the ~ limits of the 95% confidence interval.

Does the effectiveness of polychemotherapy correlate with age (or menopausal status) of the patient?

Polychemotherapy appears more effective in younger patients.
The youngest patients had the greatest degree of benefit from polychemotherapy (Table 2). There was a general trend to less benefit in older patients receiving adjuvant chemotherapy. There were relatively few patients older that 70 who participated in the studies (n=609), and for this older age category there was no statistically significant benefit, but the broad uncertainty interval did not rule out the possibility that these patients benefited as much as other patients older than 50.

For women who were less that 50 at the time of randomization, the effect of polychemotherapy on the risk of recurrence or death was approximately the same in pre- and perimenopausal women as in postmenopausal women in this age group (Table 3). However, the low number of young postmenopausal women made the comparative effectiveness of chemotherapy in this group uncertain. Again there were no statistically significant difference in effectiveness of therapy based of menopausal status for the subset of women from 50-69 years of age, but the was some uncertainty about the comparative effectiveness because of the low number of pre- and perimenopausal women in this age group.

Because age and menopausal status are closely related, and because there are relatively few women in some of the subsets it was difficult to determine the influence of the two factors on the effects or chemotherapy. However, overall the results suggested that age is at least as important as menopausal status in defining the amount of benefit to be obtained from polychemotherapy.

Table 2: Proportional Risk Reduction of Adverse Outcome
For Patients Treated with Polychemotherapy: Effects of Age

Age (years)	N=	% Proportional Risk Reduction (standard error)	
		Recurrence	Death
< 40	694/675	37 (7)	27 (5)
40-49	1629/1531	34 (5)	27 (5)
50-59	3362/3411	22 (4)	14 (4)
60-69	3394/3413	18 (4)	8 (4)
≥ 70	307/302	NS	NS
Overall	9386/9332	24 (2)	15 (2)

Table 3: Proportional Risk Reduction of Adverse Outcome
For Patients Treated with Polychemotherapy: Effects of Menopause

	N=	% Proportional Risk Reduction (standard error)	
Age < 50 years		Recurrence	Death
Pre-/Peri-Menopausal	2105/1959	34 (4)	27 (5)
Post-Menopausal	227/249	44 (13)	28 (15)
Age 50-69 years			
Pre-/Peri-Menopausal	710/759	24 (7)	19 (8)
Post-Menopausal	6077/6094	20 (3)	10 (3)

Does Polychemotherapy confer benefit for both Node Negative (NN) and Node Positive (NP) patients?

Yes, and to the same proportional degree.

In the Overall analysis, a complex time dependent analysis was used to address this question. This analysis found no differences between the proportional risk reductions afforded by adjuvant polychemotherapy in NN and NP subsets of patients. Incidentally this analysis showed that the greatest impact on *recurrence* from adjuvant chemotherapy occurred in the first 5 years with a smaller benefit noted after 5 years. Proportional *mortality* reductions were of similar magnitude in years 0-5 and after 5 years follow-up.

Is polychemotherapy effective in both ER positive and ER negative patients?

Yes and there is some suggestion that it is more effective in ER negative patients.

The question of whether ER-negative patients benefit from polychemotherapy was addressed by the Overview analysis (Table 4). Among women less than 50 years old there was a clear benefit in terms of reduction in the risk of recurrence and mortality conferred by polychemotherapy in both ER-positive and ER-poor patients. There was a trend to greater benefit in ER-poor (negative) patients, but this difference did not reach statistical significance.

Among women 50-69 years old there was a clear benefit conferred by polychemotherapy in terms of reduction in the risk of recurrence and mortality in both ER-positive and ER-poor patients. However, in terms of recurrence, ER-poor patients were almost twice as likely to benefit compared to ER-positive patients, and this difference was statistically significant. The magnitude of this effect was similar for mortality, but was not statistically significant.

Table 4: Proportional Risk Reduction of Adverse Outcome
For Patients Treated with Polychemotherapy: Effects of Estrogen Receptor

Estrogen Receptor		% Proportional Risk Reduction (standard error)	
		Recurrence	Death
<50 yr		35 (4)	27 (5)
ER-poor	710/688	40 (7)	35 (9)
ER-positive	565/550	33 (8)	20 (10)
50-69 yr		20 (3)	11 (3)
ER-poor	1647/1593	30 (5)	17 (6)
ER-positive	3359/3434	18 (4)	9 (5)

Does the use of an anthracycline improve polychemotherapy?

Yes, but the proportional and absolute amount is modest.
The question of whether anthracyclines have improved chemotherapeutic regimens has been addressed in 11 trials involving patients who were randomized between anthracycline- and non-anthracycline-containing adjuvant polychemotherapy regimens. Anthracycline-containing regimens did appear to be superior to CMF-like regimens lacking anthracyclines (Table 5). Patients receiving anthracycline-containing regimens were afforded a significant reduction in recurrence and marginally significant reduction in mortality. The absolute difference in overall mortality rate at 5 years was 3% (p=0.02).

The question of how much benefit anthracyclines add is still uncertain since the follow-up in many of these trials is short. Also in these trials about 70% of the women were premenopausal, leaving the question open as to whether anthracyclines have different levels of effectiveness in pre- and post-menopausal women.

Table 5. Proportional Risk Reduction of Adverse Outcome for Patients Treated with Adjuvant Anthracycline vs Non-Anthracycline Regimens

	N=	% Proportional Risk Reduction (standard error)	
Regimen		Recurrence	Death
With anthracyclines vs without	3477/3473	12 (4)	11 (5)

Are the shorter regimens as effective as the more prolonged regimens?

Yes, a shortening of regimens to 6 months or less has been accomplished without a major reduction in the effectiveness of adjuvant polychemotherapy.
The question of the optimal length of adjuvant chemotherapy treatment has been addressed in 11 trials included in the Overview analysis (Table 6). These trials compared a regimen given for different durations. In general, there was a slight trend suggesting that regimens administered for a longer duration were associated with a greater reduction in risk of recurrence, but this small difference did not translate into a survival advantage. Overall this analysis suggests that general reduction in the duration of the adjuvant polychemotherapy regimens have been accomplished without sacrificing efficacy.

Table 6. Proportional Risk Reduction of Adverse Outcome for Patients Treated with Longer vs Shorter Regimens

	N=	% Proportional Risk Reduction (standard error)	
Regimen		Recurrence	Death
Longer vs Shorter	3049/3055	7 (4)	-1 (5)

Is polychemotherapy effective in patients who also get adjuvant tamoxifen?

Yes, for postmenopausal patients this is clear. For premenopausal patients it is probable, but there is still some uncertainty.

Because of the relatively few premenopausal patients who participated in the polychemotherapy plus tamoxifen vs tamoxifen trials, there are wide confidence intervals about the effectiveness of polychemotherapy in these women (Table 7). Therefore although among women less than 50 years old there was no statistically significant difference in the effectiveness of chemotherapy between patients who did or who did not receive adjuvant tamoxifen, a difference could not be ruled out.

Among women 50-69 years old there was a clear benefit, in terms of reduction in the risk of recurrence and mortality, conferred by polychemotherapy in both patients who did or who did not receive additional adjuvant tamoxifen. The magnitude of this addition benefit appears not to be affected by whether the adjuvant tamoxifen was also administered.

Table 7. Proportional Risk Reduction Afforded by Polychemotherapy of Adverse Outcome for Patients Treated With or Without Adjuvant Tamoxifen

		% Proportional Risk Reduction (standard error)	
		Recurrence	Death
<50 years old		35 (4)	27 (5)
C + tam vs tam	340/300	21 (13)	25 (14)
C vs nil	1992/1908	37 (4)	28 (5)
50-69 years old		20 (3)	11 (3)
C + tam vs tam	4582/4610	19 (3)	11 (4)
C vs nil	2205/2243	22 (4)	12 (4)

Is polychemotherapy safe, and does it confer long-term net health benefits?

Yes

At ten years of follow-up patients who received adjuvant polychemotherapy did not have an excess of non-breast cancer related mortality. There was a small decrease in the risk of second breast cancers (Table 8). The rate of non-breast cancer related deaths was actually slightly lower in the patients randomized to get chemotherapy, but not statistically significant different between the groups. This was also true in the subset of women less than 50 years of age, but the number of such deaths was low (31 vs 30). Adjuvant chemotherapy reduced the proportional risk of a second primary breast cancer by a statistically significant 20%. Although this information is reassuring, there is still uncertainty over long-term effects beyond 10 years, particularly for such subsets of women as those getting intensive anthracycline-based regimens and for women undergoing early menopause.

Table 8. Effects of Adjuvant Polychemotherapy on Non-Breast Cancer Related Mortality and the Incidence of Second Breast Cancers

	10 year risk per 1,000 Patients		Significance Difference?
	Chemo-therapy	Control	
Non-Breast cancer mortality	66	75	No
Contralateral breast cancer incidence	44	55	Yes

Given the proportional risk reduction seen for polychemotherapy, how large are the absolute risk reductions?

At ten years of follow-up, both NN and NP patients who participated in these trials experienced statistically significant absolute reductions in the risk of relapse and death.

Kaplan-Meier curves generated from the Overview analysis show that all four major subsets of patients (generated on the basis of nodal status: negative vs positive; and age: < 50 years vs 50-69 years) obtain a statistically significant reduction in relapse and death at 10 years of follow-up. These results are summarized in Table 9. For many of these scenarios the improvement is substantial. Obviously some NN patients have a much lower than average risk of a negative outcome and will achieve less absolute benefit than the average NN patient.

One of the simplifying misconceptions that arises from the Overview analysis is that one can simply calculate the absolute risk reduction by multiplying the proportional risk reduction by the risk of a negative outcome if the therapy is not given. This simplification is fairly accurate when the risk of negative outcome is well less than 50%. An illustration of the inaccuracies that can arise from this oversimplification can be demonstrated using the data from the Overview analysis. For premenopausal women the expected proportional risk reduction for recurrence is ~35%. Given the observed ~40% and ~70% risk of recurrence for NN and NP patients, respectively, this should translate into an absolute risk reduction of 14% and 24%, which is greater than the observed risk reduction of 10% and 15%. This discrepancy arises because the proportional risk reduction as calculated by the Overview statisticians is actually in terms of proportional reduction of *annual* risk (see discussion of proportional risk reduction).

Table 9. Absolute Benefit in Terms of % Risk Reduction of Adverse Outcome Afforded by Polychemotherapy

	Disease Free Survival		
	With Polychemotherapy	With No Polychemotherapy	Absolute % Benefit
<50 years			
NN	68.3%	58.0%	10.3%
NP	47.6%	32.2%	15.4%
50-69 years			
NN	65.6%	59.9%	5.7%
NP	43.4%	38.0%	5.4%

	Overall Survival		
	With Polychemotherapy	With No Polychemotherapy	Absolute % Benefit
<50 years			
NN	77.6%	71.9%	5.7%
NP	53.8%	41.4%	12.4%
50-69 years			
NN	71.2%	64.8%	6.4%
NP	48.6%	46.3%	2.3%

Are there any significant weaknesses in the Overview analysis?

Yes, but it is the best compilation of studies available.
The Overview analysis' major weakness is that it is a summary compilation of data. Its estimates of the efficacy of therapy are those for the *average* polychemotherapeutic regimen. It is probable that these estimates are slightly conservative as some of the regimens included are certainly inferior, and current therapies particularly with present supportive therapies now available are somewhat better. Nonetheless examining the results of the recently reported adjuvant chemotherapy trials in terms of proportional risk reductions shows them not to be much different than the Overview analysis results.

The point also may be raised that the Overview analysis projection of the absolute benefit might be interpreted as the percentage of patients that benefit from adjuvant polychemotherapy. The Overview analysis, however, makes no such claims. In fact, the data from the Overview analysis cannot be used to infer what percentage of patients derive at least some modest benefit from adjuvant therapy.

Finally it would have been useful if additional techniques (such as multivariate analysis) had been applied to the data rather than just the meta-analysis. Perhaps a multivariate analysis might have allowed a better appreciation of the independent contributions of the different parameters.

SUMMARY OF ADJUVANT POLYCHEMOTHERAPY

The strongest conclusion of the Overview analysis is that the proportional benefits of polychemotherapy appeared to be largely unaffected by menopausal status, nodal status, or whether adjuvant tamoxifen was also used. Polychemotherapy also conferred benefit for both ER-positive and ER-negative patients. Patients older that 50 experienced less, but still statistically significant benefit. There was insufficient data to confirm the value of adjuvant polychemotherapy for patients 70 years old or older. Anthracycline-containing adjuvant regimens seem modestly more effective that non-anthracycline-containing regimens.

It was noted, however, that these were proportional benefits, and the absolute magnitude of benefit would depend on the baseline risk of the patient, and is relatively small in patients with favorable low risk tumors.

Overall, the Overview analysis strongly supported the use of adjuvant polychemotherapy therapy but recognized that the decision to use adjuvant chemotherapy depended on a judgment balancing the projected benefit of the polychemotherapy with its costs and side effects.

PRACTICAL SUMMARY OF THE 1998 OVERVIEW

The 1998 Overview analysis shows that there are effective adjuvant strategies for women irrespective of menopausal and ER status. It suggests that these benefits occur in both NN and NP women to approximately the same degree. The results suggest that for ER-negative patients, who are at high enough risk to justify consideration of systemic adjuvant therapy, use of polychemotherapy can confer substantial benefit in both premenopausal and postmenopausal patients. The Overview's estimates are almost certainly a bit low because some regimens included in the analysis are inferior to those in widespread use today. Also the Overview analysis does not give proportional risk reductions for anthracycline-based regimens vs no therapy, so these estimates must be inferred. Since the Overview analysis estimates that anthracycline-based regimens confer an additional ~10% proportional risk reduction compared to non-anthracycline-based regimens, it might be inferred that the mortality reductions given for polychemotherapy of all trials are about 10% too low. This uncertainty is reflected in the ranges of proportional risk reductions in the table below.

The 1998 Overview analysis suggests that adjuvant tamoxifen has no benefit in ER-negative patients, and substantial benefit in ER-positive patients, irrespective of menopausal status. Thus, for ER-positive patients with a high enough risk of breast cancer-related mortality to justify consideration of systemic adjuvant therapy, tamoxifen should be part of the regimen. Because tamoxifen appeared to confer this benefit even in patients who received adjuvant chemotherapy, the most effective adjuvant therapy for ER-positive patients would appear to include both chemotherapy and tamoxifen. The Overview analysis does not provide proportional risk reductions for combined chemoendocrine therapy versus nothing, so again this must be inferred from the data. The table below shows these estimates.

Patient Subset		Preferred Adjuvant Therapy	Proportional Mortality Reduction
Premenopausal	ER -	Polychemotherapy	35-45%
	ER +	Polychemotherapy + Tam (or Tamoxifen Alone)	45 – 50% (30%)
Postmenopausal	ER-	Polychemotherapy	20-30%
	ER +	Polychemotherapy + Tam (or Tamoxifen Alone)	35 - 45% (30%)

These estimates of proportional risk reductions, combined with estimates of the risk of breast cancer related mortality can help guide decisions as to which adjuvant therapies might be appropriate for individual patients.

There are a number of as yet unanswered questions that will be addressed by future Overviews. There are intriguing early results[10] that suggest that Taxanes may add substantially (~20% additional proportional risk reduction) to the effectiveness of adjuvant chemotherapy, but whether this additional effectiveness would occur irrespective of ER or menopausal status is unclear.

REFERENCES

1. Anonymous. Effects of adjuvant tamoxifen and of cytotoxic therapy on mortality in early breast cancer: an overview of 61 randomised trials among 28,896 women. Early Breast Cancer Trialists' Collaborative Group. N Engl J Med 319:1681-1692, 1988.
2. Anonymous. Systemic treatment of early breast cancer by hormonal, cytotoxic, or immune therapy. Early Breast Cancer Trialists' Collaborative Group. Lancet 339:1-15, 71-85, 1992.
3. Anonymous. Tamoxifen for early breast cancer: an overview of randomised. Early Breast Cancer Trialists' Collaborative Group. Lancet 351: 1451-1467, 1998.
4. Ravdin PM. How can prognostic and predictive factors in breast cancer be used in a practical way today?. Recent Results in Cancer Research. 152:86-93, 1998.

5. Swedish Breast Cancer Cooperative Group. Randomized trial of two versus five years of adjuvant tamoxifen for postmenopausal early stage breast cancer. J Natl Cancer Inst 88:1543-1549, 1996.

6. Fisher B, Dignam J, Bryant J, deCillis A, Wickerham DL, Wolmark N, et al. The worth of five versus more than five years of tamoxifen therapy for breast cancer patients with negative lymph nodes and estrogen receptor-positive tumors. J Natl Cancer Inst 88:1529-1542, 1996.

7. Anonymous. Ovarian ablation in early breast cancer: An overview of randomised trials. Early Breast Cancer Trialists' Collaborative Group. Lancet 348: 1189-1196, 1996.

8. Fisher B, Costantino JP, Redmond CK, Fisher ER, Wickerham DL, Cronin WM, Bowman D, Couture J, Dimitrov NV, Evans J, Farrar W, Kavanah M, Lickley HL, Margolese R, Paterson AHG, Robidoux A, Shibata H, Terz J. Endometrial cancer in tamoxifen treated breast cancer patients: findings from the National Surgical Adjuvant Breast and Bowel Project (NSABP) B-14. J Natl Cancer Inst 86:527-537, 1994.

9. Love RR, Wiebe DA, Newcomb PA, et al. Effects of tamoxifen on cardiovascular risk factors in postmenopausal women. Ann Intern Med 115:860-864, 1991.

10. Henderson IC, Berry D, Demetri G. et al. Improved disease-free and overall survival from the addition of sequential paclitaxel but not from the escalation of doxorubicin dose level in the adjuvant chemotherapy of patients with node-positive primary breast cancer. Proc Am. Soc. Clinical Oncology 17: 390a, 1998.

9

Chemoprevention of Breast Cancer

Ruth M. O'Regan, M.D.
Instructor
Division of Hematology/Oncology
Robert H. Lurie Comprehensive Cancer Center
Northwestern University

INTRODUCTION

One in eight women in the United States will develop breast cancer. Family history, hormonal factors and benign breast disease have been identified as key factors in the development of breast cancer. Until recently the only treatment option for women identified as being at high risk of developing breast cancer was bilateral prophylactic mastectomy. Tamoxifen is the treatment of choice for patients with all stages of hormone-responsive breast cancer. Tamoxifen has a proven safety record from analysis of its use in patients with early stage breast cancer and, in postmenopausal women, it maintains bone density and lowers cholesterol levels. Lastly, tamoxifen reduces the incidence of contralateral breast cancer in women with breast cancer. Recently, in a large randomized trial where women at high risk of breast cancer were randomized to tamoxifen or placebo, tamoxifen resulted in a 50% reduction in the incidence of both invasive and non-invasive breast cancers. On the basis of this result, tamoxifen has been approved as a preventive for women at high risk of developing breast cancer. The optimum duration of tamoxifen in the preventive setting is to date unclear, but in the adjuvant setting, tamoxifen continues to have beneficial effects even after it is stopped. Tamoxifen does result in a two- to threefold increase in endometrial cancer, and new antiestrogens, such as raloxifene, are being developed to reduce this risk. The next prevention trial, called Study of Tamoxifen and Raloxifene (STAR), will randomize postmenopausal women to tamoxifen or raloxifene for five years.

A number of factors led to tamoxifen being chosen to test as a preventive agent for breast cancer. Firstly, it was established many years ago that tamoxifen can prevent breast cancer in rats.[1-5] Secondly, through tamoxifen's use as an adjuvant treatment in women with breast cancer, the drug has been established as a safe, well-tolerated therapy.[6] Lastly, tamoxifen has been shown to maintain bone density in postmenopausal women,[7,8] and reduce cholesterol levels.[9,10] Additionally, tamoxifen is known to reduce the incidence of cancer of the contralateral breast in women with breast cancer.[6] In this review, we will discuss the use of tamoxifen as a treatment and preventive for breast cancer and develop the rationale for comparing tamoxifen to raloxifene as breast cancer preventives.

RISK FACTORS FOR BREAST CANCER

Family History

Family history is a well recognized risk factor for the development of breast cancer. The majority of women with a family history do not have a genetically transmitted form of the disease. However, 5%-10% of cases are linked to inherited gene mutations. To date, two genes have been identified, BRCA 1, located on chromosome 17q21,[11] and BRCA 2, located on chromosome 13q12-13.[12] These mutations, which are inherited in an autosomal dominant manner, are associated with a lifetime risk of 50%-80% of developing breast cancer.[13,14] Patients carrying these genes are also at increased risk for developing ovarian cancer, the risk being higher for BRCA 1 carriers.[15] These genes are especially seen in women of Ashkenazi Jewish descent, and specific abnormalities of the genes are seen in these women.[14] Other inherited gene mutations, such as those in the tumor suppressor gene p53, may account for approximately 1% of breast cancer cases occurring in young women.[16,17]

The remaining 90% of women with a family history of breast cancer do not carry a gene mutation and are at significantly less risk of developing breast cancer. The risk increases with the number of first degree relatives with breast cancer but rarely exceeds 30%, much less than in women carrying a gene mutation. Factors suggesting genetically transmitted breast cancer include multiple relatives with breast cancer, family history of ovarian cancer in association with breast cancer, bilateral breast cancer and breast cancer at an early age. These patients should be referred for genetic counseling.

Hormonal Risk Factors

Breast cancer development is clearly related to exposure to endogenous hormones. Early menarche,[18] late menopause,[19] nulliparity and late age of first child[20] are risk factors for breast cancer development, probably due to an increased number of ovulatory cycles. In agreement with this physical activity in adolescence has been reported to decrease risk, possibly due to a higher rate of anovulatory cycles.[21,22] Postmenopausal obesity has been associated with an increased risk of developing breast cancer, perhaps due to increased peripheral estrogen production.[23] A number of other possible hormonal risk factors have been examined, including abortion[24,25] and duration of lactation,[26,27] but have not been found conclusively to increase the risk of breast cancer.

There appears to be no significant increase in breast cancer risk with the use of oral contraceptives.[28] Estrogen replacement therapy is associated with a small but significant increase in risk of breast cancer, but it is unclear whether duration of estrogen replacement therapy affects this increased risk.[29,30]

Overall, the increased risk of breast cancer associated with hormonal factors is low and not enough to classify a woman as high risk.

Benign Breast Disease

The standard classification of benign breast disease is divided into non-proliferative, proliferative, and proliferative with atypia. Non-proliferative breast diseases, which include fibroadenoma, metaplasia, mild hyperplasia, and cysts, are not associated with an increased risk of breast cancer. The proliferative breast diseases, papillomas and sclerosing adenosis, are associated with an increase in relative risk from 1.5 to 2.0. Lastly, the proliferative breast diseases, atypical ductal and atypical lobular hyperplasia, are associated with an increase in relative risk of between 4.5 and 5.0.[31] Proliferative breast diseases are more common in patients with mammographic abnormalities[32] and a positive family history.[33]

Lobular carcinoma in situ (LCIS) is clearly associated with an increased incidence of breast cancer, which can occur in either breast. Previously, LCIS was managed either by blind biopsies, looking for invasive cancer, or with bilateral mastectomy. Women with LCIS were eligible for the first NSABP-P1 trial, in which they were randomized to tamoxifen or placebo.

Other Risk Factors

Exposure to ionizing radiation has been clearly associated with increased risk of breast cancer,[34-36] and women treated with radiation for Hodgkin's disease should start annual mammograms at an early age. Some evidence suggests that increased dietary fat may be associated with increased breast cancer risk,[37] but recently intake of dietary fat as an adult has not been shown to increase risk.[38,39] There appears to be an association between alcohol intake and breast cancer risk, with an increase in relative risk of 1.4 for each 24g of alcohol consumed daily.[40]

Interaction Between Risk Factors

Difficulties arise in determining women at high risk because of the interaction between risk factors: women can have a number of risk factors and other factors which are known to decrease risk. The Gail model[41] was devised in an attempt to incorporate a number of risk factors for breast cancer and estimate a women's relative risk. This model takes into account number of first degree relatives with breast cancer, age of menarche, age of first live birth, and number of previous breast biopsies. For example, a 30-year-old women with menarche at 14, birth of first child at 22, and no family history of breast cancer or personal history of benign breast disease has a 8.5% lifetime risk of breast cancer. As comparison, a 30-year-old woman who had menarche at 11, is nulliparous, has two first degree relatives with breast cancer, and has had one prior breast biopsy has a 40.2% lifetime risk of developing breast cancer. Certain limitations exist including only first degree relatives with breast cancer and underestimating the increased risk associated with atypical hyperplasia. The Gail model has been used to determine women at high risk of breast cancer who are candidates for breast cancer prevention.

TAMOXIFEN AS A TREATMENT FOR BREAST CANCER

Tamoxifen is currently FDA-approved for the treatment of all stages of hormone-responsive breast cancer in women of all ages. The Overview

Analysis of adjuvant breast cancer trials demonstrates conclusively that tamoxifen prolongs disease-free and overall survival in women of all ages, both pre- and postmenopausal, with both node-positive and node-negative early stage breast cancer.[6] In both early stage and advanced breast cancer, benefit is seen in only patients with estrogen receptor-positive disease.[6]

Contralateral Breast Cancer

Women with a diagnosis of breast cancer are at at least threefold higher risk of developing cancer in the opposite breast. The 1998 Overview Analysis clearly demonstrates that tamoxifen significantly reduces this risk.[6] Reduction in risk of developing contralateral breast cancer is greater with longer durations of tamoxifen, with a 50% reduction noted following five years of tamoxifen (Figure 1).[6] This reduction in contralateral breast cancer appears to persist even after the drug is stopped.[6] Tamoxifen was approved by the FDA in 1998 for this indication.

Duration of Tamoxifen

Currently, much controversy surrounds the optimal duration of adjuvant tamoxifen for early stage breast cancer. Undoubtedly five years of tamoxifen is associated with a better outcome than two years.[6,42,43] However, it is unclear whether more than five years is better than five years. Two studies have noted a worse outcome for patients treated with more than five years, compared to five years of tamoxifen.[44,45] For this reason, the National Cancer Institute is currently recommending that women receive five years of adjuvant tamoxifen and no more. When results of the ATTOM (Adjuvant Tamoxifen-Treatment Offer More) and ATLAS (Adjuvant Tamoxifen-Longer Against Shorter) trials, both of which randomize patients to five years or longer of adjuvant tamoxifen, are available, there will be a definitive answer to the question of optimal duration of adjuvant tamoxifen. Until this question is resolved, it is unclear what duration of tamoxifen should be recommended to women receiving tamoxifen as a preventive agent.

Effect of Tamoxifen on Bones

Despite tamoxifen's antiestrogenic effects on the breast, it has partial estrogen-like effects elsewhere in the body. Therefore, although tamoxifen would be expected to reduce bone mineral density, this is, in fact, not the case. Tamoxifen maintains bone density in the ovariectomized rat.[46,47] In clinical studies in postmenopausal women, tamoxifen results in significant increases in trabecular bone density, compared with control, and produces a trend to reduced loss of cortical bone density.[7,8] Additionally, the NSABP-P1 prevention trial demonstrates a non-significant reduction of 50% in hip fractures in women treated with tamoxifen, compared with placebo.[48] Interestingly, it appears that the protective effects of tamoxifen on bone can be increased by bisphosphonate treatment. Saarto and colleagues randomized postmenopausal women with early stage breast cancer to tamoxifen, with or without the bisphosphonate, clodronate, and noted that the effects of tamoxifen on bones could be further augmented with the addition of clodronate for three years.[49] In premenopausal women, however, tamoxifen results in a slight reduction in bone mineral density.[50]

In summary, there is no evidence to suggest that tamoxifen accelerates bone loss, although a slight reduction in bone density is seen in premenopausal women, and it even appears to prevent bone loss in postmenopausal women.

Effects of Tamoxifen on Lipids and Cardiovascular Events

It is well-documented that estrogen replacement therapy is protective against coronary artery disease.[51] At least part of this protective effect is felt to be due to the effects of estrogen on the lipid profile, reducing low density lipoproteins (LDLs)[52] and increasing high density lipoprotein (HDL) levels.[53] In adjuvant breast cancer trials, tamoxifen significantly reduces total cholesterol levels, predominantly due to a reduction in LDL cholesterol.[54-56] Tamoxifen, however, either does not change or slightly increases HDL cholesterol,[55-57] suggesting that its effects on the lipid profile are not identical to estrogen. Tamoxifen also reduces fibrinogen,[56,57] lipoprotein(a),[56-58] and homocysteine,[59] all recognized risk factors for the development of coronary artery disease.

Therefore, it would be expected that tamoxifen will protect against coronary heart disease in a similar manner to estrogen. Overall, however, the data are not conclusive. A 25% reduction in cardiovascular mortality was noted in the 1992 Overview Analysis.[60] The Swedish adjuvant trial noted a reduction in hospital admissions due to cardiac disease, but no definite decrease in coronary heart disease, in tamoxifen-treated patients.[61] The Scottish group noted a significant reduction in fatal myocardial infarctions in patients treated with tamoxifen for five years compared with control.[62] The NSABP-B14 trial noted a non-significant trend toward reduced myocardial infarctions with five years of tamoxifen.[63]   However, no significant reduction in myocardial infarction rate or in rate of coronary artery bypass or angioplasty was found in the NSABP-P1 prevention trial.[48] In summary, to date there is no clear evidence that tamoxifen reduces the incidence of coronary heart disease, which may be partly explained by the fact that no women at high risk for coronary heart disease were entered in the adjuvant studies. More importantly, however, there is no evidence that tamoxifen increases the risk of coronary heart disease.

Tamoxifen and Endometrial Cancer

A major concern with tamoxifen use in the treatment, and now in the prevention, of breast cancer has been the finding that it is associated with an increased incidence of endometrial cancer through its partial estrogenic effects on the uterus.   Review of the literature, however, demonstrates that the risk of endometrial cancer is only increased two- to threefold with tamoxifen.[6,64] Additionally, despite one study to the contrary,[65] tamoxifen is associated with endometrial tumors of low grade and stage and a good prognosis.[48]   The majority of endometrial tumors associated with tamoxifen occur after short durations of therapy, and therefore, it seems likely that tamoxifen, rather than causing endometrial cancer, is actually stimulating the growth of preexisting endometrial cancer.

TAMOXIFEN AS A BREAST CANCER PREVENTIVE

There are four reasons to advance with testing tamoxifen as a breast cancer preventive. First, tamoxifen has been shown to prevent the development of breast cancer in animals. Second, through the adjuvant studies, tamoxifen was found to have an excellent safety profile. Third, tamoxifen has been shown to have target-site specific actions around the body, maintaining bone density and improving the lipid profile. Lastly, tamoxifen had been shown to protect against the development of contralateral breast cancer in women with a diagnosis of breast cancer.

Animal Studies

It has been recognized for some time that tamoxifen prevents the development of breast tumors in rats, induced by certain toxins, including dimethylbenzanthracene(DMBA), N-nitrosomethylurea (NMU), and ionizing radiation.[1-5,66]   Additionally, long-term treatment with tamoxifen prevents spontaneous carcinogenesis in C3H/OUJ mice infected with the mouse mammary tumor virus.[67]

Clinical Studies

Royal Marsden Pilot Study

The Royal Marsden Pilot Study was initiated as a toxicology study and was not designed to address the role of tamoxifen as a breast cancer preventive. However, recently the trial was analyzed for breast cancer incidence.[68]

Women at high risk of developing breast cancer were randomized to receive tamoxifen 20 mg daily for up to 8 years or placebo. Women were eligible if they had at least one first degree relative with breast cancer under age 50, a first degree relative with breast cancer at any age, or another affected first or second degree relative or a first degree relative with bilateral breast cancer. A national study is ongoing, and in the United Kingdom and Australia, an accrual of 12,000 women is planned.

In general tamoxifen was well-tolerated with high compliance rates.[69] There was a significant increase in hot flashes, especially in premenopausal women, vaginal discharge, and menstrual irregularities.[69] There was no increase in thromboembolic events between the tamoxifen and placebo-treated patients.[69] A significant decrease in cholesterol was noted early and sustained throughout the duration of treatment.[69]   In premenopausal women, tamoxifen caused a significant loss of bone in both lumbar spine and hip.[69]   In contrast, in postmenopausal women, tamoxifen significantly increased bone mineral density in the spine and hip compared with untreated women.[69] Tamoxifen increased endometrial thickness and the incidence of benign ovarian cysts.[69]

Breast cancer incidence was analyzed at 70 month follow-up[68] (Figure 2). A number of women in both arms received estrogen replacement therapy. There was no significant difference in the rate of breast cancer between the tamoxifen- and placebo-treated women.   Analysis of women on estrogen replacement therapy did not reveal an interaction with tamoxifen. To date it is unclear why no decrease in rate of breast cancer was noted in this study. It is possible that many of the women had genetically transmitted breast cancer, which may not respond to tamoxifen. Additionally, the trial may have been underpowered to demonstrate a difference between the two groups.

NSABP-P1 Trial

This prospective study was designed specifically to assess the worth of tamoxifen as a preventive agent in women at high risk of developing breast cancer. Recruitment was closed after accruing 13,388 women because the estimated risk would provide sufficient events to prove whether tamoxifen prevented breast cancer. Women were identified as high risk according to the Gail model.[41] Eligible women were those over the age of 60 or women between the ages of 35 and 59 whose risk of developing breast cancer, according to the Gail model, was equal to that of a 60-year-old woman. Additionally, any woman over the age of 35 with a diagnosis of LCIS was eligible for randomization.

Other endpoints of the study were analysis of rate of fractures and cardiovascular deaths and to establish the role of genetic markers in the etiology of breast cancer.

Results were reported after 47.7 months because the statistical significance proved the benefits of tamoxifen.[48] There was a significant reduction in invasive and non-invasive breast cancer incidence in the tamoxifen-treated patients, 124 and 239 cases in the tamoxifen- and placebo-treated patients, respectively (Figure 2). Overall, there was a 49% reduction in the rate of invasive breast cancer and a 50% reduction in the rate of noninvasive breast cancer. Women with LCIS and atypical hyperplasia had a 56% and 86% reduction in breast cancer incidence, respectively. Benefits of tamoxifen were seen in all age groups (Figure 3). Tamoxifen only reduced the incidence of ER-positive tumors and did not significantly reduce the incidence of ER-negative tumors. Tamoxifen reduced the incidence of node-positive and node-negative tumors. To date the effect of genetic markers and the rate of breast cancer prevention with tamoxifen is unavailable.

Tamoxifen resulted in a non-significant reduction in osteoporotic fractures, especially in women over the age of 50.[48] No difference in cardiovascular parameters, including rate of myocardial infarction, angina, coronary artery bypass grafting, or angioplasty, was noted between the two groups.[48] The risk of developing endometrial cancer was increased two- to threefold in women treated with tamoxifen.[48] All the tumors were of low grade and stage, and no one treated with tamoxifen died from endometrial cancer. The risk of thromboembolic disease, both deep venous thrombosis and pulmonary embolus, was increased in women taking tamoxifen, especially in women over the age of 50.[48] There was a non-significant increase in strokes in women taking tamoxifen. Additionally, there was an increase in the incidence of cataracts and cataract surgery in women taking tamoxifen.[48] Quality of life assessments between the two groups was not significantly different.[48]

Italian Trial

The third prevention study randomized women aged 35 to 70 to tamoxifen 20 mg daily or placebo. This trial was different from the other trials in that women were only eligible if they had had a hysterectomy. Eligible women were not required to be at high risk for developing breast cancer and in fact, as many had had premenopausal oopherectomies. They were at a low risk of developing breast cancer. Additionally, the study was closed prematurely because of poor recruitment and compliance. Although 5,408 women were randomized, 1,422 withdrew and only 149 completed five years of treatment. There was no significant difference in the rate of breast cancer between the two groups, 19 and 22 occurring in the tamoxifen and placebo groups, respectively[70] (Figure 2). There was a significant greater incidence of thrombophlebitis in the tamoxifen group compared with the placebo group.[70]

In summary, one large prevention trial demonstrates a significant reduction in breast cancer incidence with tamoxifen treatment[48] (Figure 2). Two smaller studies, however, do not show a significant difference in breast cancer incidence[68,70] (Figure 2). One of these trials randomized women at normal to low risk of breast cancer.[70] The other was designed as a pilot study and despite now having 90% to detect a decrease in breast cancer rate of 50%, does not show a significant difference.[68] The NSABP-P1 trial is much larger than the other trials and shows a significant reduction in breast cancer rate.[48] On the basis of this large study, tamoxifen has been approved by the FDA for the prevention of breast cancer in high risk women. One important question that remains to be answered is how long tamoxifen should be continued as a preventive. Five years is the current recommendation based on the data from adjuvant trials, where the effects of tamoxifen in reducing contralateral breast cancer persist even after the drug is stopped. Future trials will compare tamoxifen with other newer antiestrogens in an effort to identify an agent that is safer than tamoxifen, particularly in regard to endometrial cancer incidence.

SELECTIVE ESTROGEN RECEPTOR MODULATION

Selective estrogen receptor modulators (SERMs) are drugs which, like tamoxifen, have target site specific actions around a woman's body, acting as an estrogen in certain tissues and an antiestrogen in others. The molecular mechanisms underlying this target site specificity are to date unclear. The ideal SERM (Figure 4) will act as an antiestrogen in the breast and endometrium but as an estrogen in bone, liver (improving the lipid profile), and central nervous system (reducing the incidence of hot flashes). Therefore, tamoxifen is not ideal since it acts as an estrogen on the endometrium, increasing the incidence of endometrial cancer, and as an antiestrogen in the central nervous system.

Raloxifene is a SERM which, like tamoxifen, acts as an antiestrogen on the breast but as an estrogen on bones and on the lipid profile. To date, it appears to be less estrogenic in the human uterus than tamoxifen.

Effects on Breast Cancer

In the rat, raloxifene inhibits the growth of DMBA-induced mammary carcinomata, although tamoxifen is more potent.[71] Additionally, like tamoxifen, raloxifene prevents the growth of NMU-induced breast tumors in rats.[5,72] Raloxifene inhibits the growth of breast cancer cells in culture.[73,74]

There is limited data on the use of raloxifene as a treatment for advanced breast cancer. One trial in patients with heavily pretreated advanced breast cancer demonstrated no responses.[75] Another small study in previously untreated patients showed a 30% response rate in patients receiving raloxifene at 300 mg daily.[76]

Effects on Bones

In ovariectomized mice, raloxifene maintains bone density.[46,77-80] At high doses, raloxifene has similar effects to estrogen on markers of bone turnover.[81] A large study, in which postmenopausal women were randomized to placebo or to treatment with three different doses of raloxifene, demonstrated a significant increase in bone density in the lumbar spine and in the hip.[82] Increases in bone density seen was similar for women receiving 60 mg of raloxifene compared with the higher doeses.[82] Therefore, raloxifene is approved at a dose of 60 mg a day for the prevention of osteoporosis in postmenopausal women.

Effects on Lipids

Like tamoxifen, raloxifene reduces the level of total cholesterol by reducing LDL cholesterol but has no effect on HDL cholesterol levels.[82]   It is unclear, however, if raloxifene reduces the incidence of cardiovascular disease. A prospective randomized trial is currently ongoing to determine if raloxifene can reduce the incidence of coronary artery disease in postmenopausal women with risk factors for coronary heart disease.

Effects on the Endometrium

Raloxifene and its analogs have low estrogenic effects on the rat uterus.[83-86] Raloxifene, however, does not appear to be a complete antiestrogen in the uterus, exhibiting partial activation of estrogen-regulated genes.[87]   In women randomized to raloxifene for the prevention of osteoporosis, there was no significant difference in uterine thickness between patients receiving raloxifene compared to placebo-treated patients.[82]   In animals, raloxifene increases the growth of human endometrial cancer by half that seen with tamoxifen, suggesting that it is less estrogenic than tamoxifen.[88]   Additionally, an osteoporosis study noted a trend to reduced endometrial cancer in women treated with raloxifene compared with placebo.[89]

Raloxifene as a Breast Cancer Preventive

Two databases of placebo controlled osteoporosis trials have been analyzed to determine if raloxifene can prevent breast cancer. The Multiple Outcomes of Raloxifene Evaluation (MORE) trial randomized 7,704 postmenopausal women with osteoporosis to placebo or raloxifene at 60 mg and 120 mg daily. At two years, there is a highly significant reduction of 70% in breast cancer incidence in the raloxifene-treated patients compared with those treated with placebo[89] (Figure 2).   The second database analyzed all placebo-controlled trials and includes 10,553 women. At three years, there is a significant 54% reduction in the incidence of breast cancer in raloxifene-treated patients compared with placebo[90] (Figure 2). Like tamoxifen, only the rate of ER-positive tumors was reduced.[90]

Study of Tamoxifen and Raloxifene (STAR)

On the basis of the results of the NSABP-P1 trial,[48] the NSABP has begun a second prevention trial in which postmenopausal women at high risk of developing breast cancer will be randomized to receive tamoxifen 20 mg or raloxifene 60 mg daily for five years (Figure 5). The primary aim of this trial is to determine if raloxifene reduces the incidence of invasive breast cancer in women at high risk. Secondary endpoints include a comparison of the two drugs' effects on the bones, the lipid profile, and general toxicities. It will be important to see whether raloxifene, unlike tamoxifen, does not increase the incidence of endometrial cancer. Women in this trial will have routine screening for endometrial cancer, i.e., an annual pelvic examination, and will not have annual endometrial biopsies. Premenopausal women are currently not eligible for the STAR trial as there is no data on the effects of raloxifene on bones in these women. The National Cancer Institute is currently examining the effects of raloxifene on bones in premenopausal women and depending on the results, premenopausal women may be eligible later. Results for the STAR trial should be available by 2006.

CONCLUSION

Tamoxifen has been extensively used in the treatment of breast cancer and has been established as a safe agent with beneficial effects on bones and lipids. Based on a large randomized trial in which tamoxifen reduced the incidence of invasive breast cancer by 50%, tamoxifen is now approved for the prevention of breast cancer in postmenopausal women at high risk of developing breast cancer. Tamoxifen is, however, associated with an increased risk of endometrial cancer, and newer agents are being examined to reduce this risk. Raloxifene is one such agent, which appears less estrogenic than tamoxifen on the endometrium. For this reason, the current prevention trial randomizes postmenopausal women at high risk for breast cancer to five years of tamoxifen or raloxifene.

REFERENCES

1.   Jordan VC: Antitumor activity of the antioestrogen ICI 46,474 (tamoxifen) in the dimethylbenzanthracene (DMBA)-induced rat mammary carcinoma model. J Steroid Biochem 1974;5:354.

2.   Jordan VC: Effects of tamoxifen (ICI 46,474) on initiation and growth of
      DMBA-induced rat mammary carcinomata. Eur J Cancer 1976;12:419-
      424

3.   Jordan VC, Allen KE: Pharmacology of tamoxifen in laboratory animals.
      Cancer Treat Rep 1980;64:745 –759.

4.   Jordan VC, Allen KE: Evaluation of the anitumour activity of the
      nonsteroidal antioestrogen monohydroxytamoxifen in DMBA-induced rat
      mammary carcinoma model. Eur J Cancer 1980;16:239-251.

5.   Gottardis MM, Jordan VC: The antitumor actions of keoxifene
      (raloxifene) and tamoxifen in the N_nitromethylurea-induced rat
      mammary carcinoma model. Cancer Res 1987;47:4020-4924.

6.   Early Breast Cancer Trialists' Collaborative Group. Tamoxifen for early
      breast cancer: an overview of the randomized trials.   Lancet
      1988;351:1451-1467.

7.   Love RR, Mazess RB, Barden HS, Epstein S, Newcomb PA, Jordan VC,
      Carbone PP, DeMets DL. Effects of tamoxifen on bone mineral density in
      postmenopausal women with breast cancer. N Engl J Med 1992;326:852-
      856.

8.   Kristensen B, Ejlertsen B, Dalgaard P, Larsen L, Holmegaard SN,
      Transbol I, Mouridsen HT.   Tamoxifen and bone metabolism in
      postmenopausal low-risk breast cancer patients: A randomized study. J
      Clin Oncol 1994;12:992-997.

9.   Love RR, Wiebe DA, Feyzi JM, Newcomb PA, Chappell RJ. Effects of
      tamoxifen on cardiovascular risk factors in postmenopausal women after
      five years of treatment. J Natl Cancer Inst 1994;86:1534-1539.

10.   Rossner S, Wallgren A: Serum lipoproteins and proteins after breast
      cancer surgery and effects of tamoxifen. Atherosclerosis 1984;52:339-
      346.

11.   Miki Y, Swen J, Shattuck-Eidens D, et al: A strong candidate for the
      breast and ovarian cancer susceptibility gene. Science 1994;265:66-71.

12.   Wooster R, Neuhausen SL, Mangion J, et al: Localization of a breast
      cancer susceptibility gene, BRCA 2, to chromosomes 13q12-13. Science
      1994;265:2088-2090.

13.   Easton DF, Bishop DT, Ford D, et al: Genetic linkage analysis in familial
      breast and ovarian cancer: results from 214 families. Am J Hum Genet
      1993;52:678-701.

14.   Struewing JP, Hartge P, Wacholder S, et al: The risk of cancer associated
      with specific mutations of BRCA1 and BRCA2 among Ashkenasi Jews.
      N Engl J Med 1997;336:1401-1408.

15. King MC, Rowell S, Love SM: Inherited breast and ovarian cancer. What are the risks ? What are the choices ? JAMA 1993;269:175-180.
16. Malkin D, Li FP, Strong LC, et al: Germ line p53 mutations in a familial syndrome of breast cancer, sarcomas and other neoplasms. Science 1990;250:1233-1238.
17. Sidrensky D, Tokino T, Helzlsouer K; Inherited p53 mutation in breast cancer. Cancer Res 1992;52:2984-2989.
18. MacMahon B, Trichopoulos D, Brown J, et al: Age of menarce, probability of ovulation and breast cancer risk. Int J Cancer 1982;29:13-16.
19. Trichopoulos D, MacMahon B, Cole P: Menopause and breast cancer risk. J Natl Cancer Inst 1972;48:605-613.
20. MacMahon B, Cole P, Lin TM, et al: Age of first birth and breast cancer risk. Bull WHO 1970;43:209-221.
21. Frisch RE, Gotz-Welbergen AV, McArthur JW, et al: Delayed menarche and amenorrhea of college athletes in relation to age of onset of training. JAMA 1981;246:1559-1563.
22. Bernstein L, Henderson BE, Hanisch R, et al: Physical exercise and reduced risk of breast cancer in young women. J Natl Cancer Inst 1994;86:1403-1408.
23. De Waard F, Baanders-van Halecijn E: A prospective study in general practice on breast cancer risk in postmenopausal women. Int J Cancer 1974;14:153-160.
24. Harris BM, Eklund G, Meririk O, et al: Risk of cancer of the breast after legal abortion during the first trimester: A Swedish register study. Br J Med 1989;299:1430-1432.
25. Melbye M, Wohlfahrt J, Osen JH, et al: Induced abortion and the risk of breast cancer. N Engl J Med 1997;336:81-85.
26. Layde PM, Webster LA, Baughman AL, et al: The independent associations of parity, age at first fullterm pregnancy, and duration of breast feeding with the risk of breast cancer. J Clin Epidemiol 1989;42:963-973.
27. Kvale G, Heuch I: Lactation and a reduced risk of premenopausal breast cancer. N Engl J Med 1994;330:81-87.
28. Malone KE, Daling JR, Weiss NS: Oral contraceptives in relation to breast cancer. Epidemiol Rev 1993;15:80-97.
29. Steinberg KK, Thacker SB, Smith SJ, et al: A meta-analysis of the effect of estrogen replacement therapy on the risk of breast cancer. JAMA 1991;265:1985-1990.

30. Sillero-Arenas M, Delgado-Rodriquez M, Rodriquez-Canteras R, et al: Menopausal hormone replacement therapy and breast cancer: a meta-analysis. Obstet Gynecol 1992;79:286-294.

31. Jordan VC, Morrow M: Tamoxifen, raloxifene and the prevention of breast cancer. Endocrine Rev 1999;20:253-278.

32. Duponmt WD, Page D: Risk factors for breast cancer in women with proliferative breast disease. N Engl J Med 1985;312:146-151.

33. Skolnick MH, Cannon-Albright LA, Goldgar DE, et al: Inheritance of proliferative breast disease in breast cancer kindreds. Science 1990;250:1715-1720.

34. Land CE, McGregor DH: Breast cancer incidence among atomic bomb survivors: implication for radiobiologic risk at low doses. J Natl Cancer Inst 1979;62:17-20.

35. Hildreth NG, Shore RE, Dvoretsky PM: The risk of breast cancer after irradiation of the thymus in infancy. N Engl J Med 1989;321:1281-1285.

36. Miller AB, Howe GR, Sherman GJ, et al: Mortality from breast cancer after irradiation during fluoroscopic examinations in patients being treated for tuberculosis. N Engl J Med 1989;321:1285-1289.

37. Armstrong B, Doll R: Environmental factors and cancer incidence and mortality in different countries with special reference to dietary practices. Int J Cancer 1975;15:617-625.

38. Hunter DJ, Willett WC: Dietary factors. In Harris JR, Lippman ME, Morrow M, Hellman S (eds.) Diseases of the Breast. Lippincott-Raven, Philadelphia, PA, pp 201-212.

39. Hunter DJ, Spiegelman D, Adami HO, et al: Cohort studies of fat intake and the risk of breast cancer – a pooled analysis. N Engl J Med 1996;334:356-361.

40. Longnecker MP, Berllin JA, Orza MJ, et al: A metaanalysis of alcohol consumption in relation to breast cancer risk. JAMA 1988;260:652-656.

41. Gail MH, Brinton LA, Byar DP, et al. Projecting individualized probabilities of developing breast cancer from white women who are being examined annually. J Natl Cancer Inst 1989;88:1543-1549.

42. Swedish Breast Cancer Cooperative Group. Randomized trial of two versus five years of adjuvant tamoxifen for postmenopausal early stage breast cancer. J Natl Cancer Inst 1996;88:1543-9.

43. Current Trials Working Party of the Cancer Research Campaign Breast Cancer Trials Group. Preliminary results from the Cancer Research Campaign Trial evaluating tamoxifen duration in women aged fifty years or older with breast cancer. J Natl Cancer Inst 1996;88:1834-9.

44.   Fisher B, Dignam J, Bryant J, et al. Five versus more than five years of tamoxifen therapy for breast cancer patients with negative lymph nodes and estrogen receptor-positive tumors. J Natl Cancer Inst 1996;88:1529-42.

45.   Stewart HJ, Forrest AP, Everington D, et al. Randomized comparison of 5 years of adjuvant tamoxifen with continuous therapy for operable breast cancer. Br J Cancer 1996;74:297-299.

46.   Jordan VC, Phelps E, Lingren JU: Effects of antiestrogens on bone in castrated and intact female rats. Breast Cancer Res Treat 1987;10:31-35.

47.   Turner RT, Wakley GK, Hannon KS, et al: Tamoxifen prevents the skeletal effects of ovarian hormone definciency in rats. J Bone Miner Res 1987;2:449-456.

48.   Fisher B, Costantino JP, Wickerham DL, et al. Tamoxifen for prevention of breast cancer: report of the National Surgical Adjuvant breast and Bowel Project P-1 Study. J Natl Cancer Inst 1998;90:1371-1388.

49.   Saarto T, Blomquist C, Valimaki M, et al. Clodronate improves bone mineral density in postmenopausal breast cancer patients treated with adjuvant antiestrogens. Br J Cancer 1997;75:602-5.

50.   Powles TJ, Hickish T, Kanis JA, et al. Effect of tamoxifen on bone mineral density measured by dual-energy x-ray absorptiometry in healthy premenopausal and postmenopausal women. J Clin Oncol 1996;14:78-84.

51.   Stampfer MJ, Colditz GA, Willett WC, et al. Postmenopausal estrogen therapy and cardiovascular disease. Ten year followup from the Nurse's Health Study. N Engl J Med 1991;325:756-762.

52.   Sacks FM, Walsh BW. Sex hormones and lipoprotein metabolism. Curr Opin Lipidol 1994;5:236-240.

53.   Nabulsi AA, Folsom AR, White A, et al. Association of hormone-replacement therapy with various cardiovascular risk factors in postmenopausal women. The Atherosclerosis Risk in Communities Study Investigators. N Engl J Med 1993;328:1069-1075.

54.   Bruning PF, Bonfrer JM, Hart AA, et al. Tamoxifen, serum lipoproteins and cardiovascular risk. Br J Cancer 1988;58:497-499.

55.   Grey AB, Stapleton JP, Evans MC, Reid IR. The effect of the anti-estrogen tamoxifen on cardiovascular risk factors in normal postmenopausal women. J Clin Endocrinol Metab 1995;80:3191-3195.

56.   Love RR, Wiebe DA, Feyzi JM, et al. Effects of tamoxifen on cardiovascular risk factors in postmenopausal women after five years of treatment. J Natl Cancer Inst 1994;86:1534-1539.

57.   Saarto T, Blomquist C, Ehnholm C, Taskinen MR, Elomaa I. Antiatherogenic effects of adjuvant antiestrogens: A randomized trial

comparing the effects of tamoxifen and toremifene on plasma lipid levels in postmenopausal women with node-positive breast cancer. J Clin Oncol 1996;14:429-433.

58.   Shewmon DA, Stock JL, Abusamra LC, Kristan MA, Baker S, Heiniluoma KM. Tamoxifen decreases lipoprotein(a) in patients with breast cancer. Metabolism 1994;43:531-532.

59.   Anker G, Lonning PE, Ueland PM, Refsum H, Lien EA. Plasma levels of the atherogenic amino acid homocysteine in postmenopausal women with breast cancer treated with tamoxifen. Int J Cancer 1995;60:365-368.

60.   Early Breast Cancer Trials Collaborative Group. Systemic therapy of early breast cancer by hormonal, cytotoxic and immune therapy: 133 randomized trials involving 331,000 recurrances and 24,000 deaths among 75,000 women. Lancet 1992;339:1-15.

61.   Rutqvist LE, Mattsson A. Cardiac and thromboembolic morbidity among postmenopausal women with early stage breast cancer in a randomized trial of adjuvant tamoxifen. J Natl Cancer Inst 1993;85:1398-1406.

62.   McDonald CC, Stewart HJ. Fatal myocardial infarction in the Scottish adjuvant tamoxifen trial. The Scottish Breast Cancer Committee. BMJ 1991;303:435-437.

63.   Costantino JP, Kuller LH, Ives DG, Fisher B, Dignam J. Coronary heart disease mortality and adjuvant tamoxifen therapy. J Natl Cancer Inst 1997;89:776-82.

64.   Assikis VJ, Neven P, Jordan VC, Vergote I. A realistic clinical perspective of tamoxifen and endometrial carcinogenesis. Eur J Cancer 1996;32A:1464-1476.

65.   Magriples U, Naftolin F, Schwartz PE, Carcangiu ML. High-grade endometrial carcinoma in tamoxifen treated breast cancer patients. J Clin Oncol 1993;11:485-490.

66.   Welsch CW, Goodrich-Smith M, Brown CK, et al: Effect of an estrogen antagonist (tamoxifen) on the initiation and progression of radiation-induced mammary tumors in female Sprague Dawley rats. Eur J Cancer 1981;17:1255-1258.

67.   Jordan VC, Lababidi MK, Langan-Fahey S: Supression of mouse mammary tumorgenesis by long-term tamoxifen therapy. J Natl Cancer Inst 1991;83:492-496.

68.   Powles TJ, Eeles E, Ashley SE, et al. Interim analysis of the incident breast cancer in the Royal Marsden Hospital tamoxifen randomized prevention trial. Lancet 1998;362:98-101.

69.   Powles TJ, Jones AL, Ashley SE, et al: The Royal Marsden Hospital pilot
       tamoxifen chemoprevention trial. Breast Cancer Res Treat 1994;31:73-
       82.
70.   Veronesi U, Maissonneuve P, Costa A, et al. Prevention of breast cancer
       with tamoxifen: preliminary findings from the Italian randomized trial
       among hysterectomised women. Lancet 1998;352:93-97.
71.   Clemens JA, Bennett DR, Black LJ, et al: Effects of the new antiestrogen
       keoxifene LY 156758 on growth of carcinogen-induced mammary tumors
       and on LH and prolactin levels. Life Sci 1983;32:2869-2875.
72.   Anzano MA, Peer CW, Smith JM, et al: Chemoprevention of mammary
       carcinogenesis in the rat: combined use of raloxifene and 9-cis-retinoic
       acid. J Natl Cancer Inst 1996;88:123-125.
73.   Poulin R, Meraud Y. Porrier D, et al: Antiestrogenic properties of
       keoxifene, trans 4-hydroxytamoxifen and ICI 164,380, a new steroidal
       antiestrogen, in ZR-75-1 human breast cancer cells. Breast Cancer Res
       Treat 1989;14:65-76.
74.   Jiang SY, Parker CJ, Jordan VC: A model to describe how a point
       mutation of the estrogen receptor alters the structure function relationship
       of antiestrogens. Breast Cancer Res Treat 1993;26:139-147.
75.   Buzdar AU, Marcus C, Holmes F, et al: Phase II evaluation of LY
       156758 in metastatic breast cancer. Oncology 1988;45:344-345.
76.   Gradishar WJ, Glusman JE, Vogel CL, et al. Raloxifene HCL, a new
       endocrine agent, is active in estrogen receptor positive (ER+) metastatic
       breast cancer. Breast Cancer Res Treat 1997;46;53 (Abs 209).
77.   Black LJ, Sato M, Rowley ER, et al: Raloxifene (LY 139,481 HCL)
       prevents bone loss and reduces serum cholesterol without causing uterine
       hypertrophy in ovariectomized rats. J Clin Invest 1994;93:63-69.
78.   Sato M, McClintock C, Kim J, et al: Dual energy x-ray absorbiometry of
       raloxifene effects on lumbar vertebrae and femora of ovariectomized rats.
       J Bone Miner Res 1994;9:715-724.
79.   Sato M, Kim J, Short LL, et al: Longitudinal and cross sectional analysis
       of raloxifene effects on tibiae from ovariectomized rats. J Pharmacol Exp
       Ther 1995;272:1252-1259.
80.   Turner CH, Sato M, Bryant HU: Raloxifene preserves bone strength and
       bone mass in ovariectomized rats. Endocrinology 1994;135:2001-2001.
81.   Draper MW, Flowers DE, Huster WJ, et al: Effects of raloxifene (LY
       139,481 HCL) on biochemical markers of bone and lipid metabolism in
       healthy postmenopausal women. In: Christiansen C, Rii S (eds)
       Proceeding 4th International Symposium on Osteoporosis and Concensus

Development Conference, Aalborg, Denmark, Handelstrykkeriet, Aalborg Aps, Denmark, pp 119-121, 1993.

82.   Delmas PD, Bjarnason NH, Mitlak BH, et al. Effects of raloxifene on bone mineral density, serum cholesterol concentrations, and uterine endometrium in postmenopausal women. N Engl J Med 1997;337:1641-1647.

83.   Jones CD, Jevnikar MG, Pike AJ, et al: Antiestrogens 2: Structure-activity studies in a series of 3 aroyl-2-arylbenzo[b]thiophene derivatives leading to [6-hydroxy-2-(4-hydrotyphenyl) benzo[b]thiene-3-yl] [4-[2-(1-piperidinyl) ethoxy-phenyl] methanone hydrochloride (LY 156758), a remarkably effective estrogen antagonist with only minimal estrogenicity. J Med Chem 1984;27:1057-1066.

84.   Black LJ, Jones CD, Falcone JF: Antagonism of estrogen action with a new benzothiphene derived antiestrogen. Life Sci 1983;32:1031-1036.

85.   Black LJ, Goode RL: Uterine bioassay of tamoxifen, trioxifene and a new estrogen antagonist (LY 117018) in rats and mice. Life Sci 1980;26:1453-1458.

86.   Jordan VC, Gosden B: Inhibition of the uterotropic activity of antiestrogens by the short acting antiestrogen LY 117018. Endocrinolgy 1983;113:463-468.

87.   Jordan VC, Gosden B: Differential antiestrogen action on the immature rat uterus: a comparison of hydroxylated antiestrogens with high affinity for the estrogen receptor. J Steroid Biochem 1983;19:1249-1258.

88.   Gottardis MM, Ricchio ME, Satyaswaroop PG, et al: Effect of steroidal and non-steroidal antiestrogens on the growth of a tamoxifen-stimulated human endometrial carcinoma (EnCa101) in athymic mice. Cancer Res 1990;50:3189-3192.

89.   Cummings SR, Eckert S, Krueger KA, et al: The effects of raloxifene on the risk of breast cancer in postmenopausal women: results form the MORE randomized trial. Multiple Outcomes of Raloxifene Evaluation. JAMA 1999;281:2189-2197.

90.   Jordan VC, Glusman JE, Eckert S, et al: Incident primary breast cancers are reduced by raloxifene: integrated data from multicenter, double-blind, randomized trials in ~ 12,000 postmenopausal women. Proc ASCO Abs 1998;466;122a.

Figure 1. Incidence of Contralateral Breast Cancer Depending on Duration of Tamoxifen in the 1998 Overview Analysis[6]

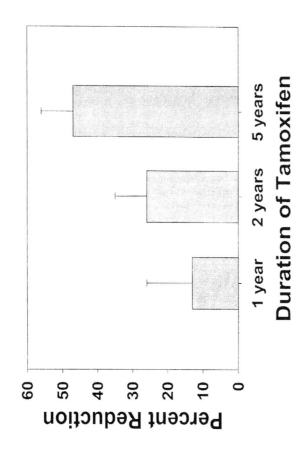

Figure 2. Comparison of Effects of Tamoxifen in the Three Breast Cancer Prevention Trials and Raloxifene in the Osteoporosis Databases[90]

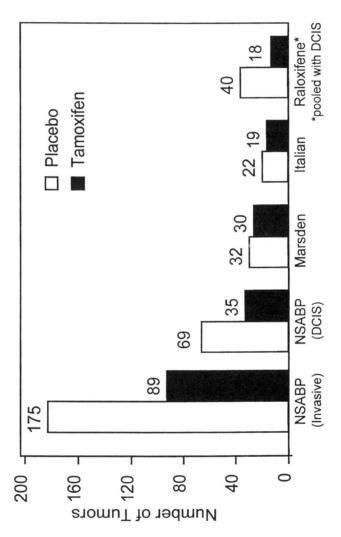

Figure 3. Tamoxifen Reduces the Incidence of Breast Cancer in All Age Groups in the NSABP-P1 Prevention Trial[48]

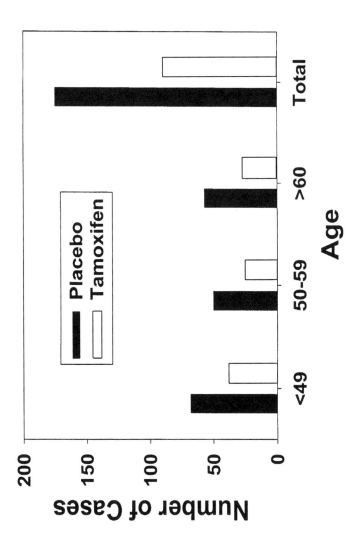

Figure 4. Effects of the Ideal Selective Estrogen Receptor Modulator (SERM)

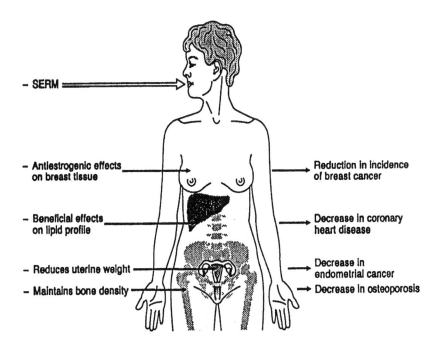

- SERM

- Antiestrogenic effects on breast tissue
- Beneficial effects on lipid profile
- Reduces uterine weight
- Maintains bone density

Reduction in incidence of breast cancer
Decrease in coronary heart disease
Decrease in endometrial cancer
Decrease in osteoporosis

Figure 5.   The STAR Trial Will Randomize Postmenopausal Women at High Risk of Breast Cancer to Tamoxifen or Raloxifene

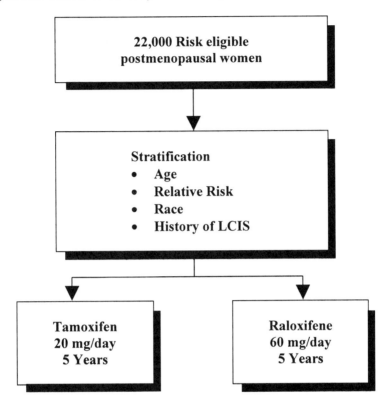

Index